ORANGA

MENTAL HEALTH MATTERS

Erin Steel

Published by Spectrum Education Limited
Lower Hutt, New Zealand
info@spectrumeducation.com

ISBN 978-1-0670169-9-9

Copyright © Spectrum Education 2024
© Erin Steel 2024

Designed and typeset by Spectrum Education, New Zealand
All photographs taken by Erin Steel

All rights reserved. No part of this publication may be reproduced, stored in a retrieval system, or transmitted in any form or by any means (electronic, mechanical, photocopying or otherwise), without the prior written permission of both the copyright owner and the publisher of this book.

Contents

2. Oranga - Overview
3. A Guide for Kaiako
5. About the Author
7. An Open Letter
9. Five Ways to Wellbeing
11. A-Z of the Five Ways to Wellbeing
20. Five Ways to Wellbeing with Your Whānau
22. Daily Focus and Motivation - Monday to Friday
27. A Gift from Focus Fit
31. Mindfulness Month
32. Food for Thought
33. Inspiring Reflection and Discussion
34. End of Term Reflection
35. Poem
38. Smart Goals
39. Developing Effective Habits
42. Revamp Your Health + Physical Education Curriculum
45. Talking Stems
48. Play Prompts
49. Strengthen Confidence
51. Whakawhetai Gratitude
52. Dare to Dream Bigger by Carrie Brightwell
55. Inspiration and Motivation by Megan Gallagher
57. Tēna koutou katoa
59. Acknowledgements
60. Testimonials

Oranga-Overview

Confidence is a powerful force. When we are armed with it, we find the courage to give our best in all areas of life—whether at home, at work, or in our personal growth. Confidence in best practice, in our own abilities, and in the support networks around us allows us to thrive, adapt, and contribute meaningfully to our communities.

This pukapuka (book) is about cultivating that confidence. It offers insights into the various supports available to enhance well-being—whether through initiatives like the Mental Health Foundation's Mental Health Awareness Week, Mindfulness Month, or Move for Mental Health. It also highlights the importance of the relationships we build with colleagues who generously share their skills and aroha.

Increasing our awareness of these resources and the power of connection, this book encourages us to lean into our own confidence, embrace the help around us and live fuller, more empowered lives.

Overview of Contents

- Open Letter - a heartfelt introduction that sets the tone for the journey ahead.
- Maximising Movement: discover the power of movement in supporting mental and physical well-being. This section delves into how regular activity can boost our energy, focus and overall hauora (well-being).
- Mental Health Awareness Week
- Why Movement Matters: explore why movement is so vital for a balanced, healthy life and how it directly impacts mental health.
- Five Ways to Wellbeing & Te Whare Tapa Whā: a comprehensive look at the Five Ways to Wellbeing framework and Ta Mason Durie's Te Whare Tapa Whā model, providing practical tools to integrate these concepts into everyday life.
- Poetry: Mindfulness Month
- An invitation to slow down and be present, with mindfulness practices and exercises that can be easily incorporated into daily routines.
- Inspiration and Motivation
- Monday to Friday - Daily Focus - inspired by Meg Gallagher - a week's worth of structured activities designed to help you focus on a different aspect of well-being each day—from self-care on Monday to reflection and gratitude on Friday.
- A playful yet informative section providing an A to Z of movement-based activities, with suggestions for keeping both body and mind active.
- Whakawhetai (Gratitude) - a reflection on the power of gratitude and how fostering an attitude of thankfulness can enhance our overall sense of well-being and connection to others.

ORANGA HINENGARO: A GUIDE FOR KAIAKO

Why does mental health matter?
It strengthens hauora, for both kaiako and ākonga,
Supporting the whole being, weaving well-being into the heart of learning.
A focus on oranga creates a taiao ako—
A learning space that nurtures success,
Where ākonga grow and kaiako thrive.
Whānau tautoko—
When we open kōrero,
We build a community of support,
Where no one stands alone.
Normalise the conversation—
Encourage open kōrero,
Check in with one another,
Use words that uplift, that soften stigma,
Create a space where well-being can breathe.
Be brave enough to share—
Your pūrākau of oranga hinengaro,
Let others see your strength in vulnerability.
And in those safe spaces,
We will wānanga,
Sharing, listening, holding space for one another.
Share the tools, the pathways to support.
Resources for ākonga and hoamahi,
So that no one is without guidance.
Every day, we can support.
Incorporate oranga hinengaro into our mahi,
Use the tools, the resources at hand.
Promote self-care, lead by example,
Both for ourselves and those we teach.
Engage in learning—
Wānanga, workshops, deepen our understanding.
Create support groups, a place to kōrero,
Be involved in community,
Where awareness grows and conversations flow.
Together, we open the path—
A learning environment that supports well-being,
For kaiako and ākonga alike.

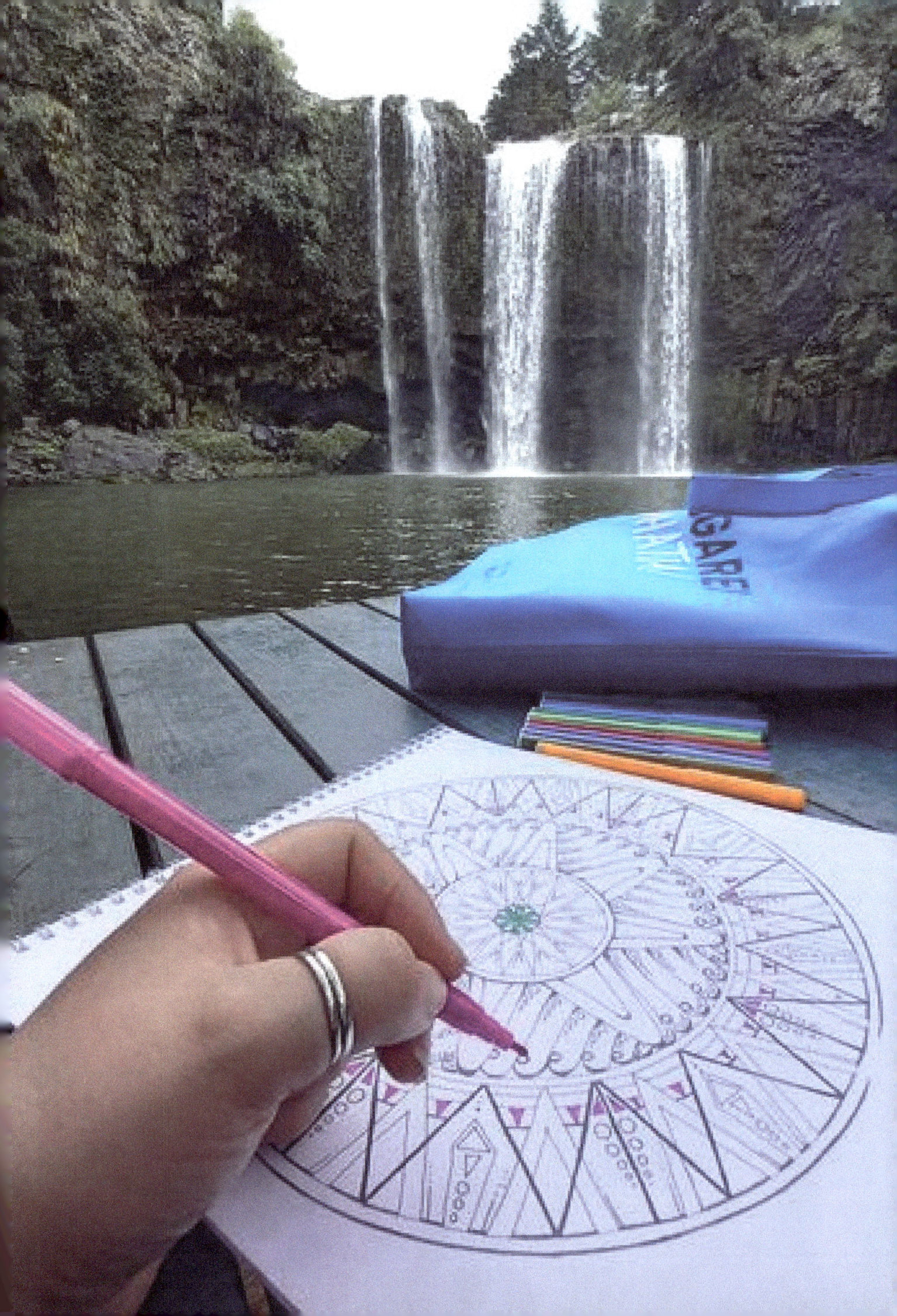

Tōku Pepeha

Kia ora e te whānau,

Nō Tāmaki Makaurau ahau,

Engari, kei Whangārei ahau e noho ana ināianei.

Ko Ngāti Kuia tōku iwi.

He kaiako ahau.

Ko Erin Steel tōku ingoa.

Nō reira, tēnā koutou, tēnā koutou, tēnā koutou katoa.

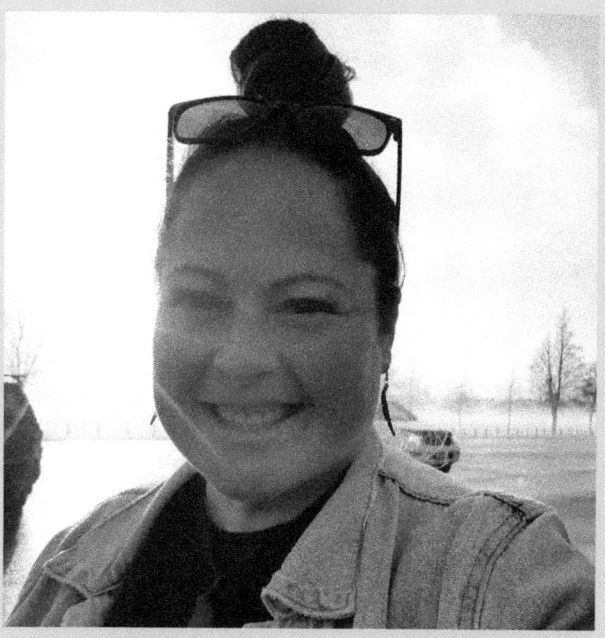

from the author

Growing up in the beautiful community of Oranga, Tāmaki Makaurau, I was surrounded by the power of connection, whānau and well-being. Oranga, a place I proudly call home, instilled in me a deep sense of belonging and the understanding of community. When we nurture our own oranga (well-being), we strengthen our ability to uplift others.

Working in education for 20 years, my journey has been educating our next generation, it's also been about supporting the well-being of kaiako and ākonga alike. I've witnessed first hand how crucial it is for kaiako to prioritise their own oranga—because when we are at our best, we can guide our hoamahi, tamariki and rangatahi to thrive.

Teaching is one of the most fulfilling and demanding roles and I've seen the extreme difference it makes when kaiako embrace practices that promote balance and joy. Whether it be through the Five Ways to Wellbeing, Te Whare Tapa Whā, or moments of mindfulness, these small but powerful actions create a positive ripple effect, feeding and supporting our classrooms and communities.

In my work across Te Tai Tokerau, I'm continually inspired by the passion of those who strive for the success of our tamariki. I am in awe of the schools that are creating supportive environments that focus on play, active recreation, sport and as a result, oranga for kaiako, ākonga and whānau.

Erin Steel

*Kaiako,
Facilitator and Coach*

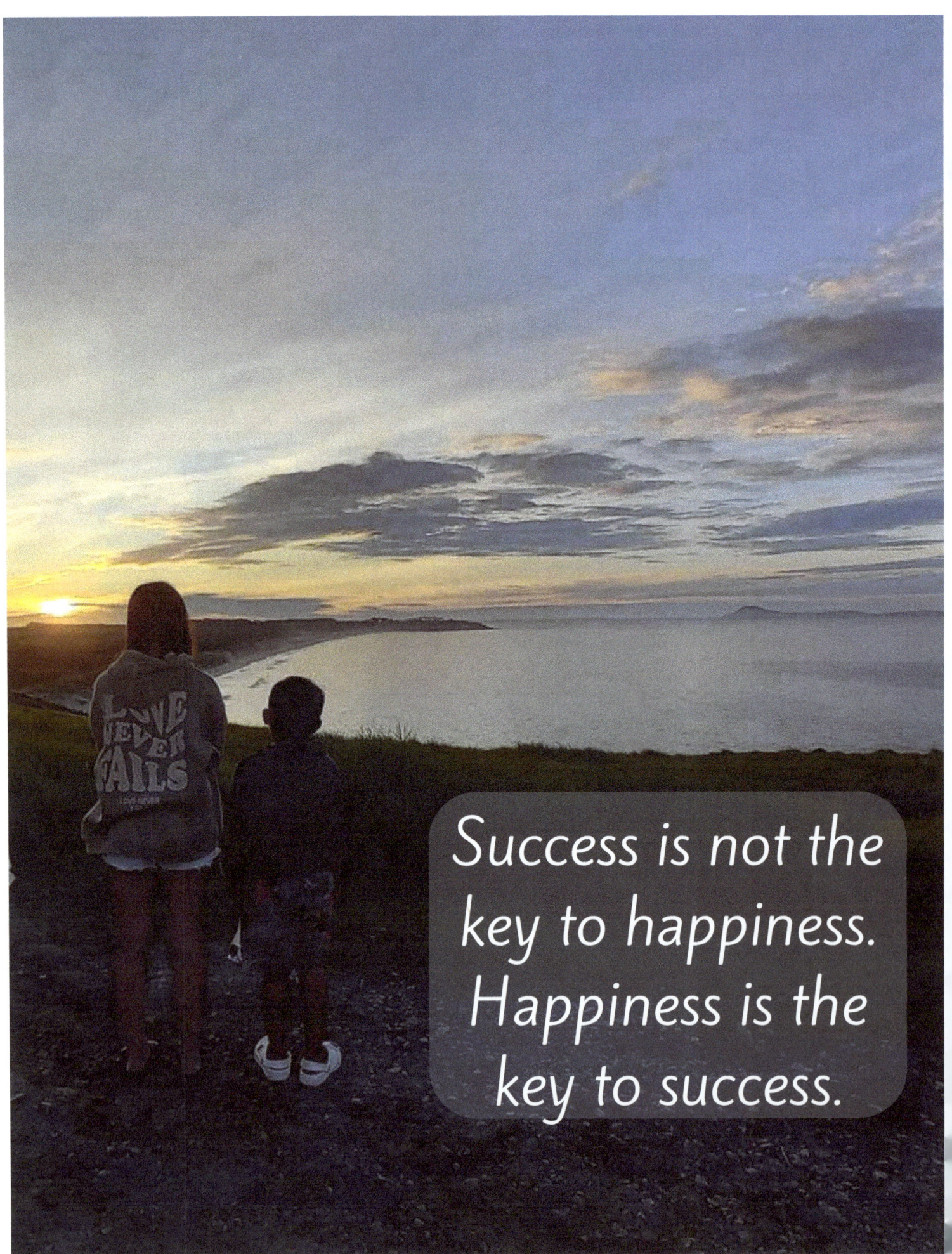

An Open Letter

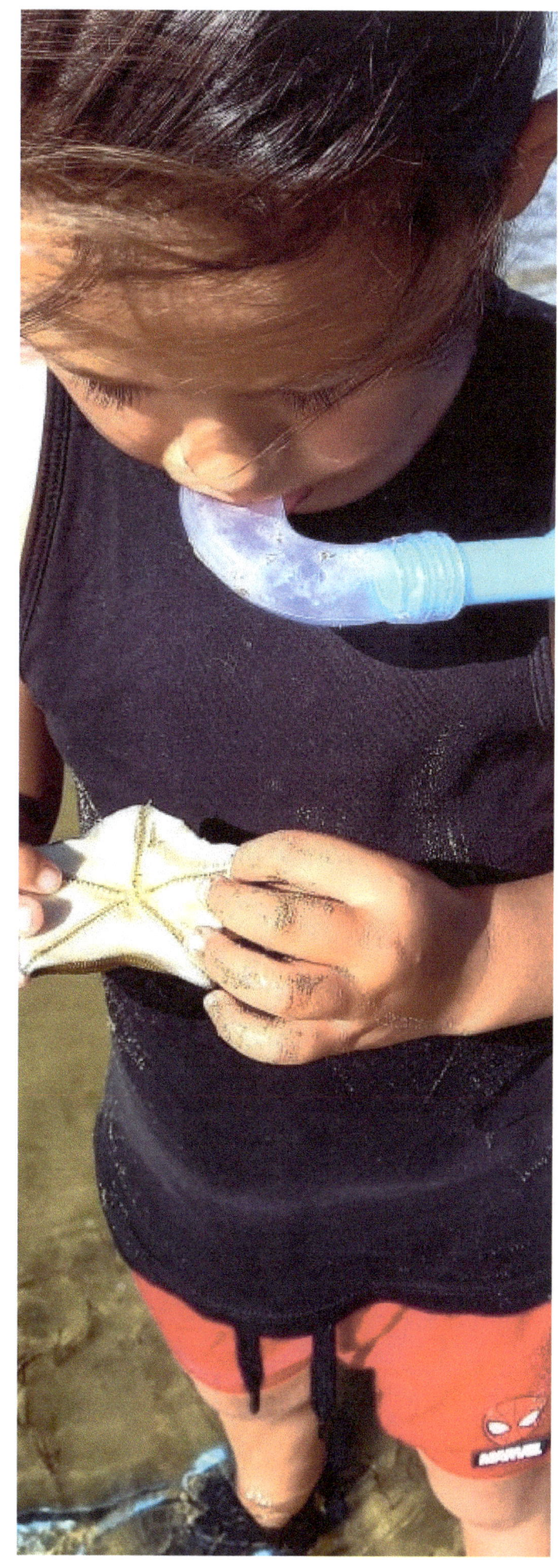

Tēnā koe,

We haven't met yet, but you are going to change our lives in ways we can't even imagine. One day, we will walk into your classroom—unsure, curious, maybe a little nervous—and you will be the person who welcomes us with a smile that instantly makes us feel safe and seen. You'll be the one who believes in us, even when we doubt ourselves. Through your patience, encouragement and kindness, we'll discover strengths we never knew we had and our confidence will grow with every lesson you share.

There will be days when we don't fully understand the world or ourselves, but you will be there—our steady guide—showing us that it's okay to stumble, to ask questions, and to try again. You'll remind us that learning is a journey and sometimes the most important lessons are the ones that come from mistakes. You'll inspire us to dream bigger, to think deeper and to push beyond what we think we're capable of.

Years from now, we may not remember every single fact or lesson, but we will never forget the way you made us feel. You will become a part of our story, someone we look back on with gratitude and warmth, knowing that it was in your classroom where we found not just knowledge, but belief in ourselves.

Thank you for choosing to be a teacher, for being our light, our guide and our champion. We may not know each other yet, but we already know one thing for sure—you are going to make a difference in our lives and we can't wait to meet you.

With hope and gratitude,
Your future students

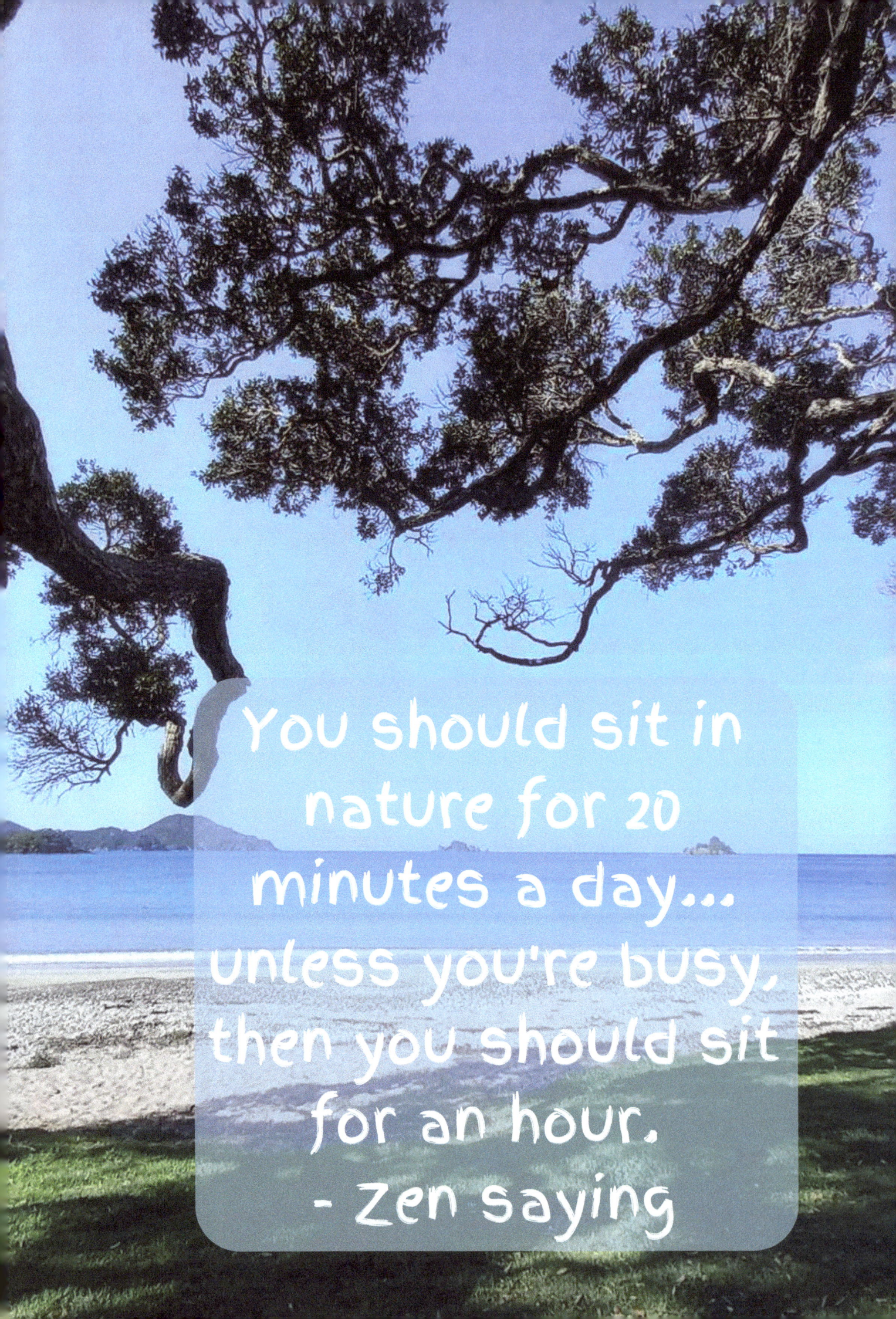

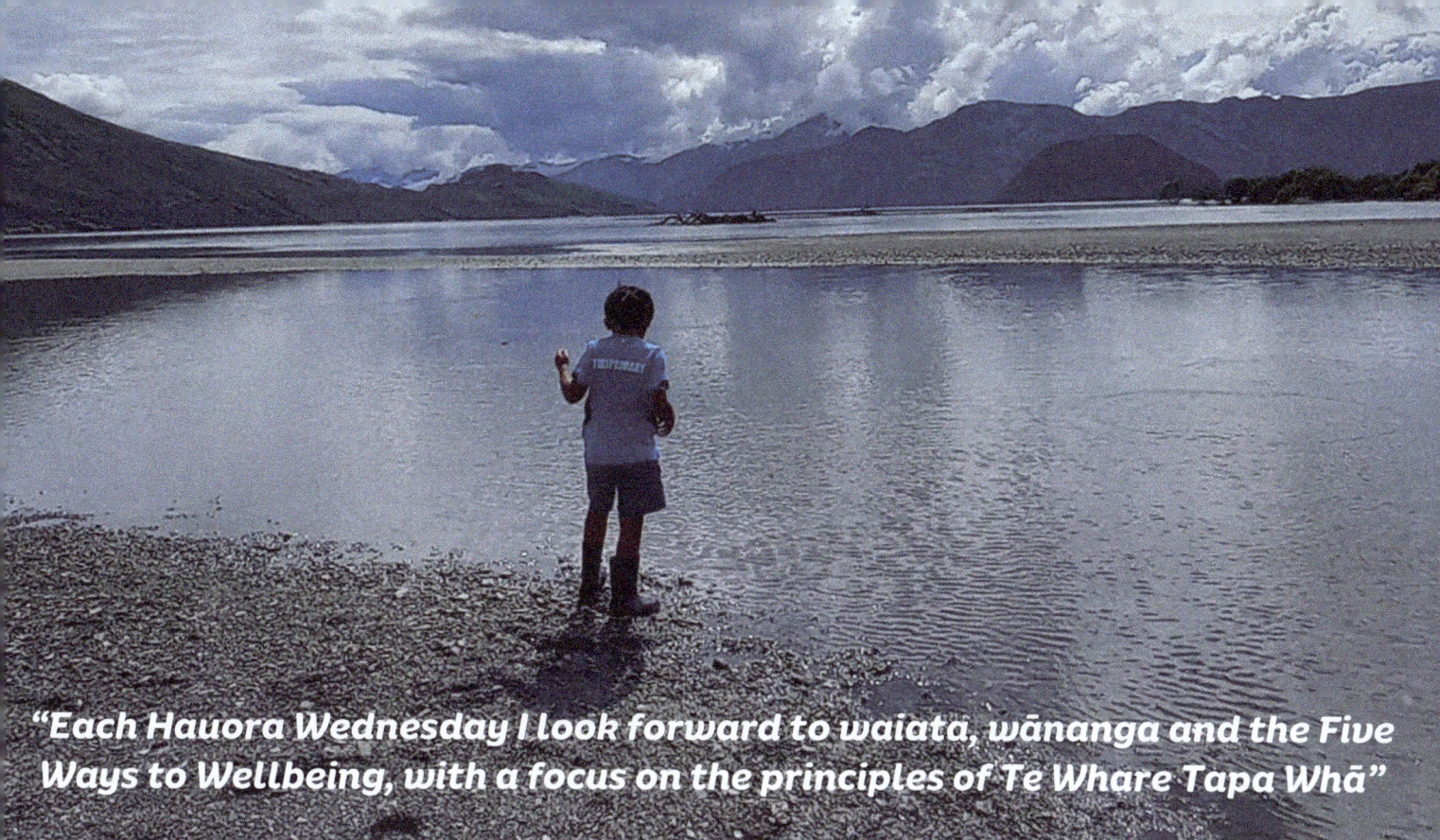

"Each Hauora Wednesday I look forward to waiata, wānanga and the Five Ways to Wellbeing, with a focus on the principles of Te Whare Tapa Whā"

Five Ways to Wellbeing

Whether applied in personal life, workplaces, or schools, the Five Ways to Wellbeing encourage intentionality in nurturing our own health and the well-being of those around us. In this article, we explore how incorporating these practices can encourage daily routines and create lasting positive change.

Taha Tinana (Physical Wellbeing) - Be Active

- Walking and talking are one of my favourite things about my mahi. Taking a brisk hīkoi during a break time or as part of a coaching catch up, together we enjoying the fresh air and sunshine or sprinkle of rain is all good to.

- This is one I struggle with the most sometimes (especially in those more stressful times) - encourage yourself to eat nutritious meals and staying hydrated throughout the day. - I don't know about you, but I find winter harder to get that wai on board... you might want to set yourself some water intake goals.

- Another suggestion could be to create a list of your favourite ways to move, use this list to learn a new jump jam, dance, sport or participate in a physical activity that you enjoy.

Taha Hinengaro (Mental and Emotional Wellbeing) - Take Notice

- Each morning I spend a few minutes practicing mindfulness or meditation to centre my thoughts. Why not give it a try and find a time that works best for you. In between hui are other opportunities to take a quick moment to find your calm.

- At the end of the day you could reflect on the positive aspects of your day and write them down or share them with a colleague.

- Taking notice of all of our emotions and finding ways to acknowledge, express and manage them - when we build our emotional intelligence, we become better equipped, able to be present and we become more able to support those around us.

Taha Whānau (Social Wellbeing) - Connect

- Reach out to a colleague, friend, or family member for a meaningful kōrero.
- Keeping in mind that that tamariki spell LOVE - T.I.M.E.
- Book yourself a recurring appointment with some of your friends each week or month.
- Organise a small group activity or coffee break to strengthen your connections with others.
- Or share a positive story or experience with your team to foster a sense of community.

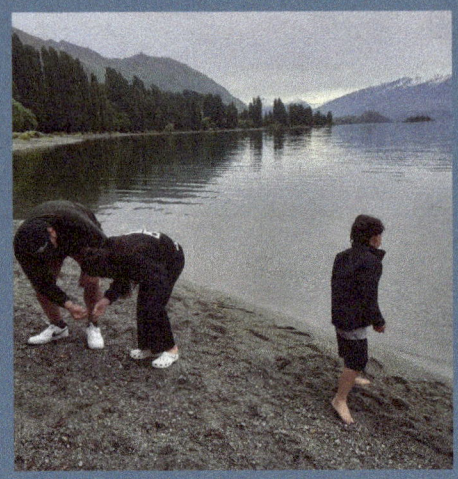

PRECIOUS WHĀNAU TIME

Taha Wairua (Spiritual Wellbeing) - Give and Keep Learning

- Engaging in activities that bring awareness and soul food to our wairua, such as spending time in nature or practicing gratitude - are just a couple of my go to tools in my kete.
- Giving back to others by offering a kind word or gesture, or by volunteering our time can also have mutual benefits.
- When was the last time you were curious about something new? Why not take some time to learn something new that enriches your sense of purpose and personal growth.

A question I ask myself most mornings before I even open my eyes - what are you doing for your wellbeing today?

I encourage you to reflect on how you are supporting your oranga using the principles of Te Whare Tapa Whā and the Five Ways to Wellbeing. Share your experiences with someone—whether it's through a photo, a short description, or a quick note about what you're doing for your wellbeing today.

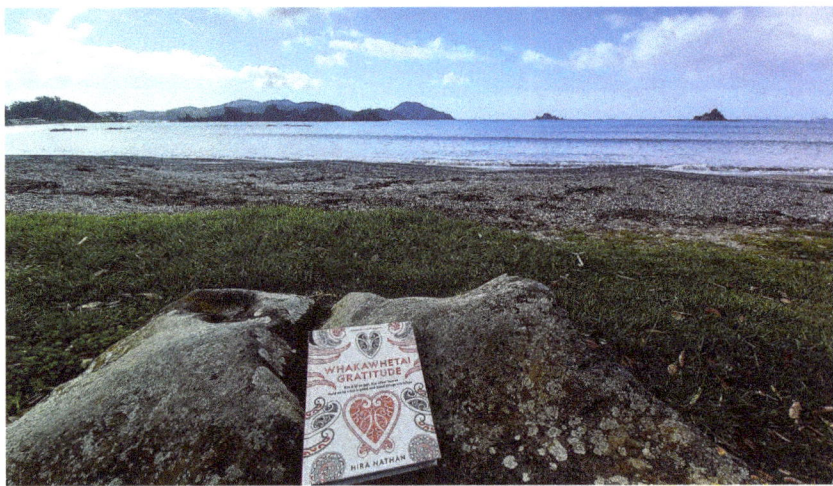

Whakawhetai Gratitude

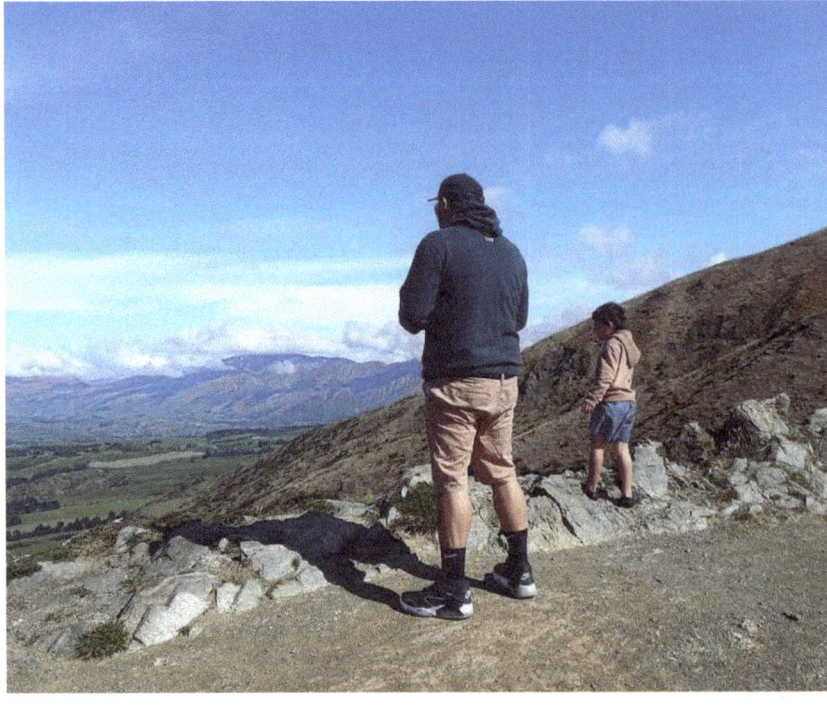

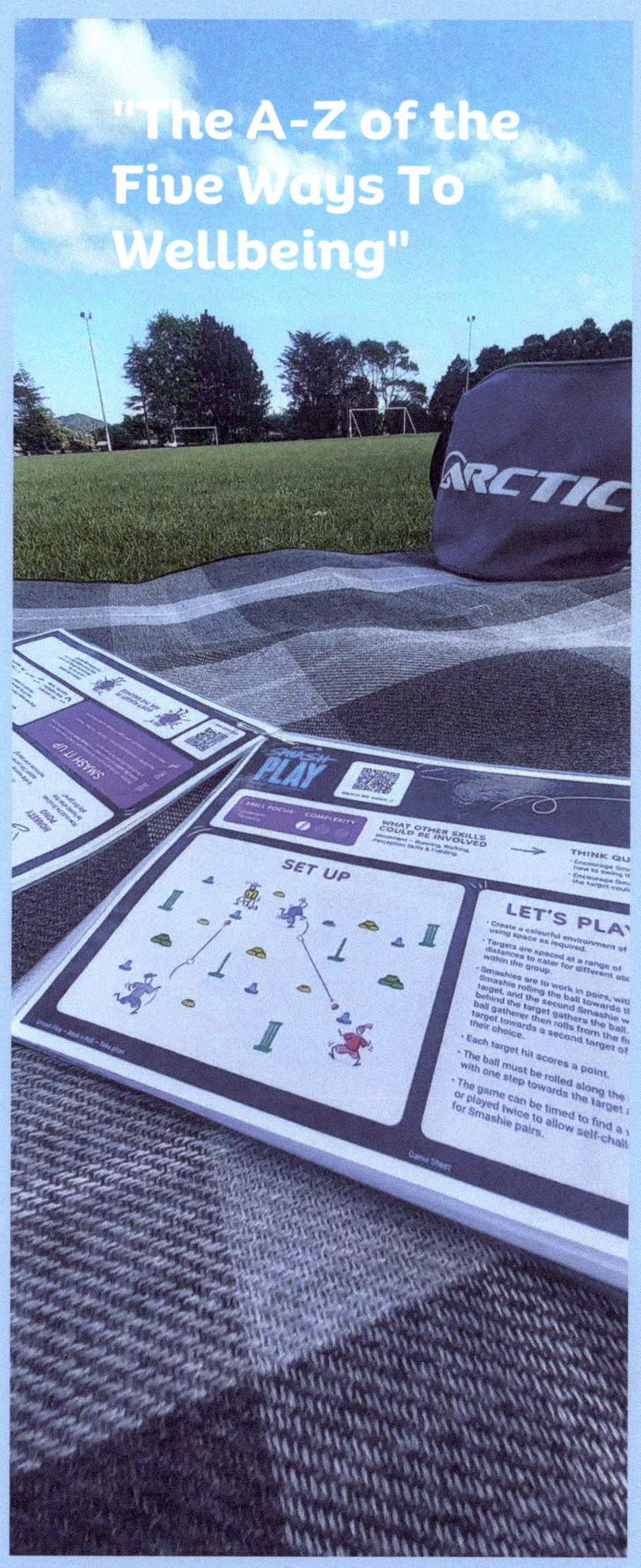

"The A-Z of the Five Ways To Wellbeing"

What do you do to protect and grow your oranga?

Teaching is one of the most fulfilling and demanding roles, and I've seen the extreme difference it makes when kaiako embrace practices that promote balance and joy. Whether through the Five Ways to Wellbeing, Te Whare Tapa Whā, or moments of mindfulness, these small but powerful actions create a positive ripple effect, nourishing our classrooms and communities.

In my work across Te Tai Tokerau, I'm continually inspired by the passion of those who strive for the success of our tamariki. Schools are creating supportive environments that focus on play, active recreation, sport and as a result oranga for kaiako, ākonga and whānau.

As you explore your own journey of oranga, consider what actions you can take to nurture your well-being so that you can continue to give your best to your whānau, your ākonga and yourself. Our oranga is a taonga— by honouring it, we uplift not only ourselves but the generations we are guiding and inspiring.

In the following pages there are plenty of ideas that you could employ to up your focus on YOU. What other ways could you bring the Five Ways to Wellbeing into focus?

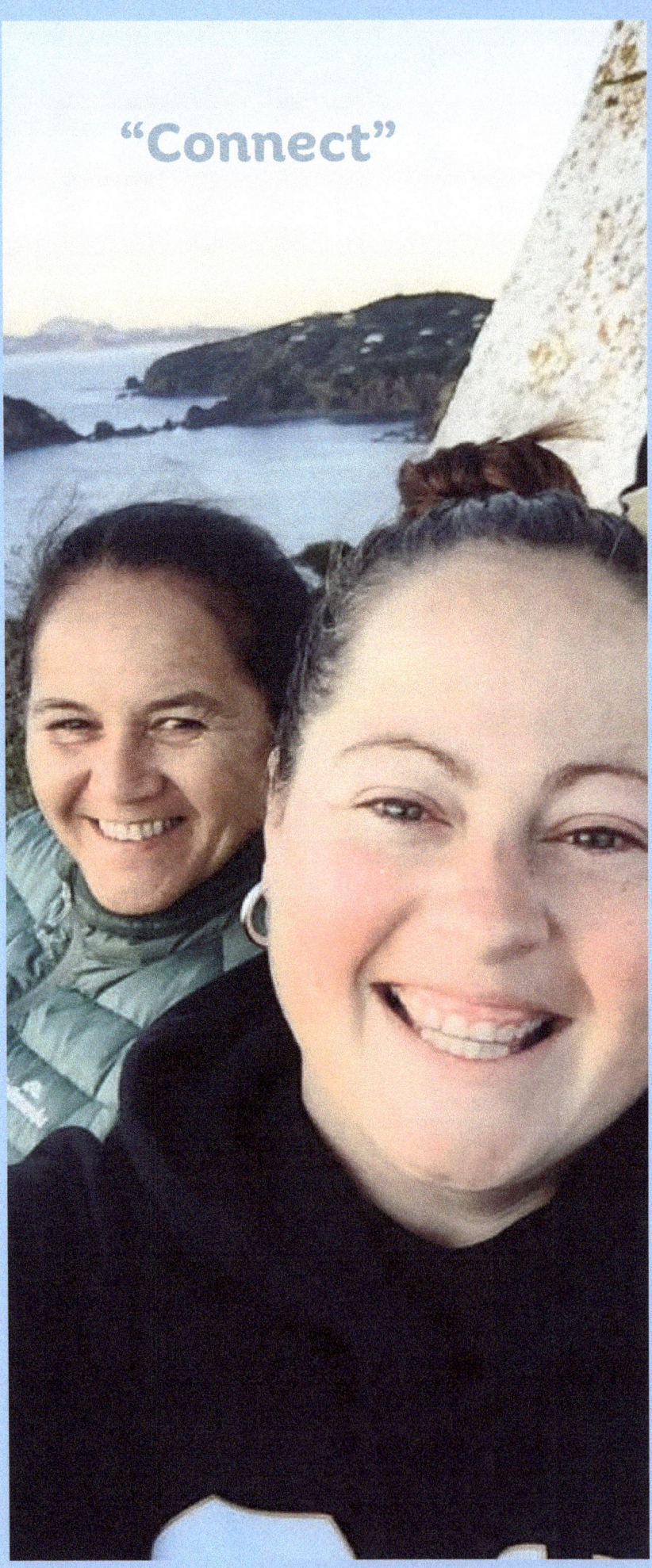

"Connect"

A - Ask someone how their day is going.
B - Be present in conversations.
C - Call a friend or whānau member just to chat.
D - Do something fun together with others.
E - Eat together as a family or team.
F - Find time for a face-to-face kōrero.
G - Go for a walk and talk with a friend.
H - Have a video call with someone far away.
I - Include others in group activities.
J - Join a club or social group.
K - Keep in touch with old friends.
L - Listen actively and show empathy.
M - Make new connections at work or in your community.
N - Notice when others need support and offer it.
O - Open up about your feelings with someone you trust.
P - Plan a social gathering or meet-up.
Q - Quiet time spent with someone can strengthen relationships.
R - Reach out to someone you haven't talked to in a while.
S - Share experiences, thoughts and ideas.
T - Text someone just to let them know you're thinking of them.
U - Unite in shared goals or activities.
V - Visit a neighbour or friend.
W - Write a letter to someone special.
X - Xtra care for relationships that matter most.
Y - Your time spent with others is valuable.
Z - Zoom in on the positive connections in your life.

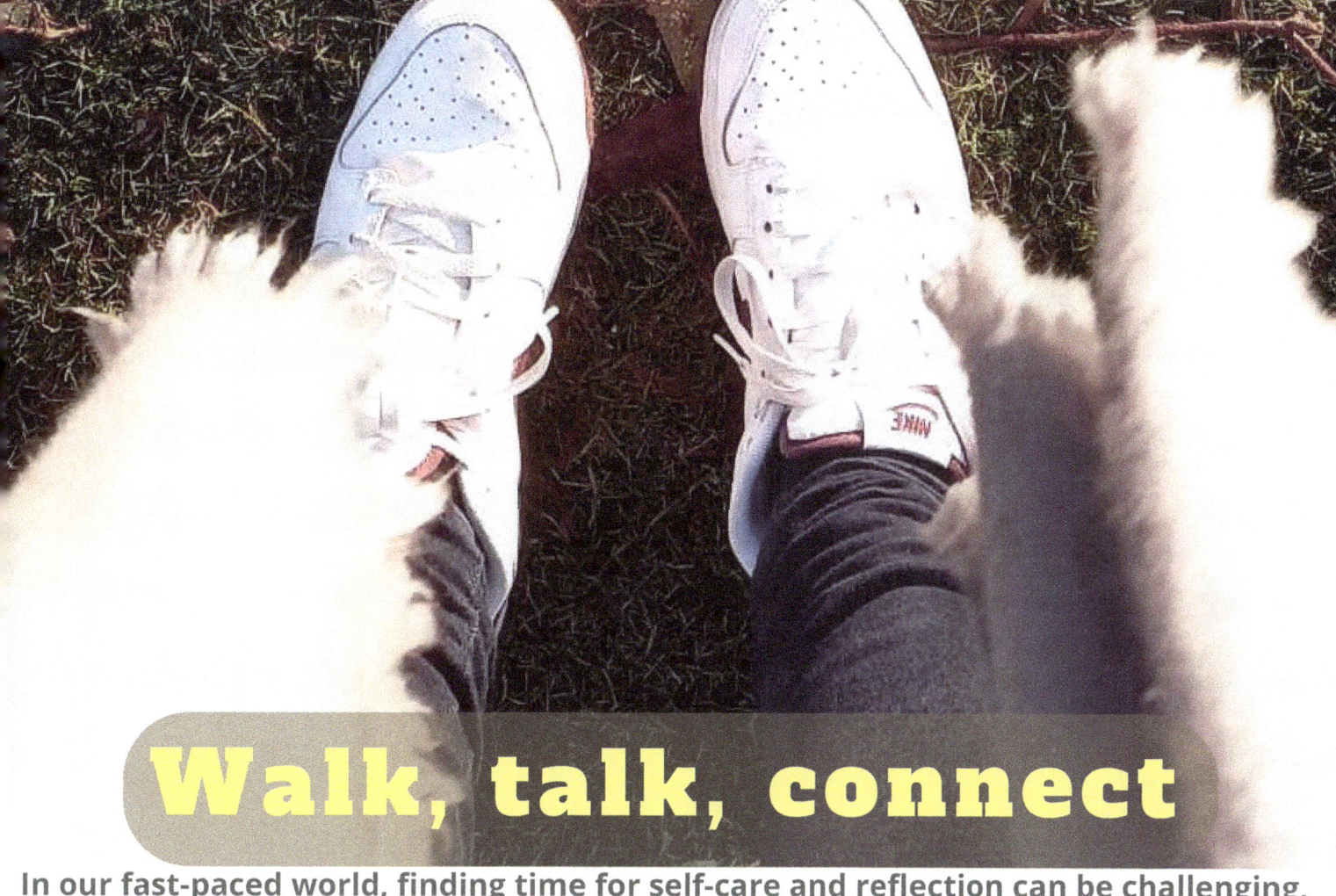

Walk, talk, connect

In our fast-paced world, finding time for self-care and reflection can be challenging, especially for those who are always giving their best to others. The simple yet profound practice of walking, talking and connecting can be a powerful tool to enhance our well-being.

Walking is more than just physical exercise; it's a way to clear your mind, reduce stress and boost your mood. Whether it's a leisurely stroll in the park or a brisk walk around your neighbourhood, taking time to move your body can help you feel more grounded and centered.

- How do you feel before and after a walk? Do you notice any changes in your mood or thoughts?
- What thoughts or insights come to mind during your walk? Are there any patterns or recurring themes?
- How can you incorporate walking into your daily routine? What are some new routes or environments you might explore?

Engaging in **meaningful conversations** with others can strengthen relationships, provide support, and offer new perspectives. Whether it's a deep discussion with a friend or a casual chat with a colleague, talking can help you process your feelings and experiences.

- How do you approach conversations when you need support or guidance? Are there ways you can improve how you communicate your needs?
- What strategies can you use to ensure your conversations are meaningful and supportive? How can you create space for open and honest dialogue?

Connection is at the heart of our well-being. Building and maintaining relationships with family, friends, and community can provide a sense of belonging and purpose. It's important to nurture these connections and find new ways to engage with others.

- What activities or experiences help you feel more connected to others? How can you make time for these in your life?
- How can you reach out to someone you haven't spoken to in a while? What steps can you take to strengthen existing relationships?

"Be Active"

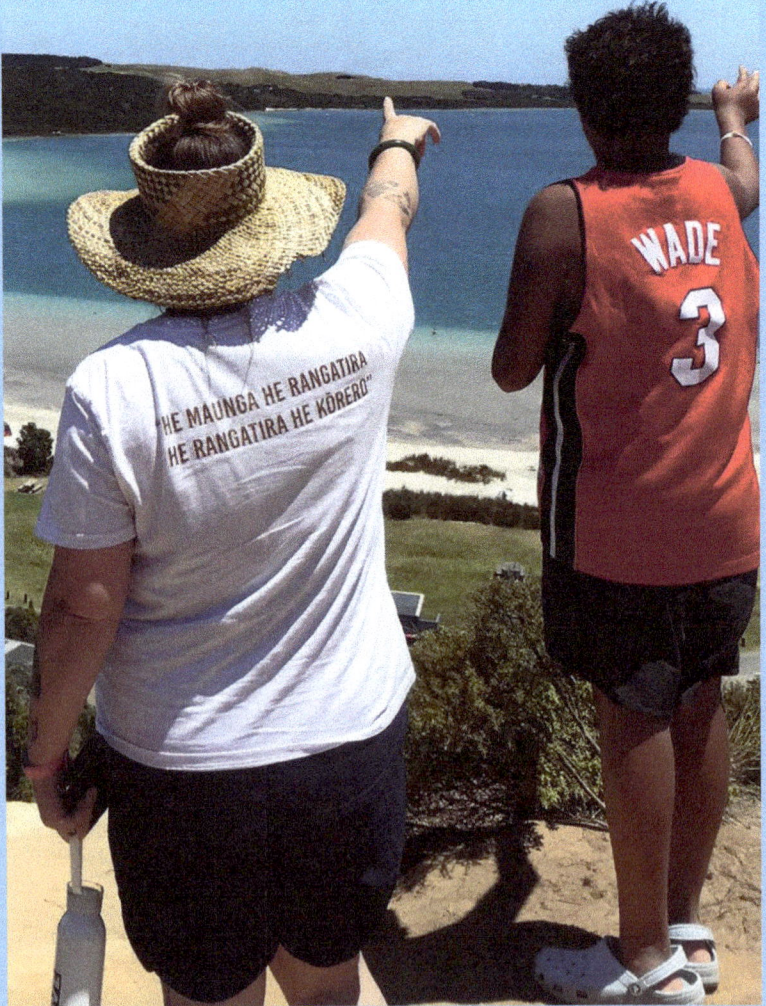

Support a colleague by inviting them to join you for a physical activity, like a walk or a quick game outside. Being active together can boost your well-being and strengthen your connection. How many other opportunities are there to engage with each other?

A - Aim to get moving every day
B - Bike ride around your neighbourhood
C - Climb a hill or staircase
D - Dance to your favorite music
E - Explore a new park or walking trail
F - Find a fun way to exercise, like sports or swimming
G - Go for a morning walk
H - Hike with friends or whānau
I - Involve yourself in group fitness classes
J - Jog or run to release stress
K - Kick a ball around with your kids or your mates
L - Lift weights or do strength exercises
M - Move during your work breaks
N - Notice how your body feels when you're active
O - Outdoor activities like gardening or beach walks
P - Play a game that gets you moving
Q - Quick stretches throughout the day
R - Ride a scooter or rollerblade
S - Swim for relaxation and exercise
T - Try a new sport or physical activity
U - Use the stairs instead of the elevator
V - Volunteer for a community event
W - Walk to your destination when possible
X - Xplore new ways to stay active
Y - Yoga to improve flexibility and mindfulness
Z - Zumba for a fun, energetic workout

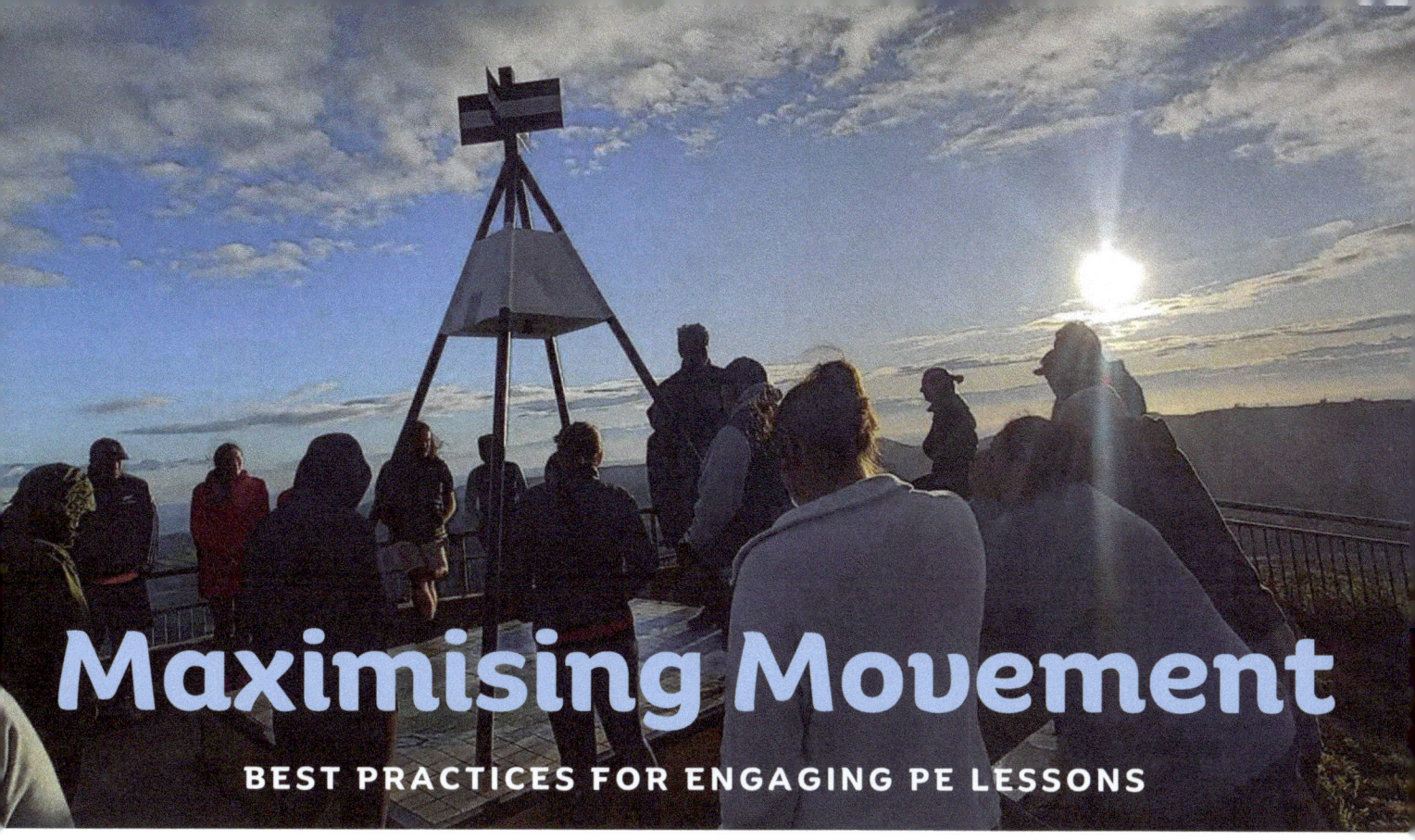

Maximising Movement
BEST PRACTICES FOR ENGAGING PE LESSONS

Clear Learning Intentions:
- Start with well-defined goals linked to the HPE curriculum so ākonga understand what they are learning and why.

Efficient Planning and Setup:
- Organise equipment and groupings before the lesson to maximise active time and minimise transitions.
- Keep instructions short and simple, using the KISS principle (Keep It Short and Simple).

Engagement and Inclusivity:
- Ensure all ākonga are actively participating by offering various roles (e.g., players, timekeepers, equipment helpers) and differentiating tasks for varying skill levels.
- Design activities that cater to all abilities, using adaptations as necessary so every ākonga can succeed.

Progression and Challenge:
- Incorporate challenges that allow ākonga to progress in skills and fitness over time, balancing the level of difficulty to maintain motivation.
- Focus on the process of learning and development rather than just the outcome.

Positive Feedback and Reinforcement:
- Give frequent, specific, and positive feedback to encourage improvement and build confidence.
- Reinforce positive behaviours like teamwork, effort and fair play to promote a supportive class culture.

Reflection and Review:
- End the lesson with a quick reflection, asking ākonga to assess their performance, how they felt and what they learned.
- Link the day's activities to broader goals like health, well-being and teamwork, making connections to life beyond PE.

Growth and Hauora:
- Encourage a growth culture by highlighting effort and improvement, not just winning or performance.
- Incorporate elements of Te Whare Tapa Whā and the Five Ways to Wellbeing to make the lesson holistic, promoting mental, social and emotional health as well as physical wellbeing.

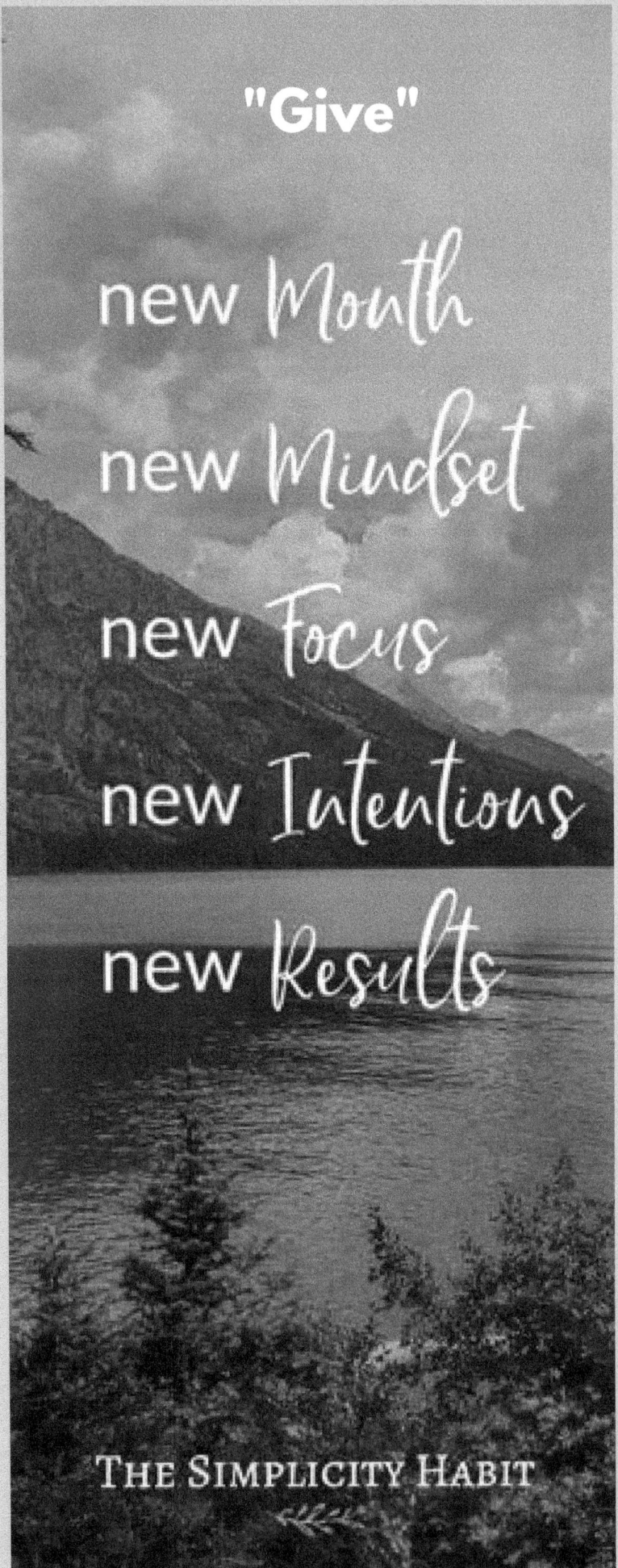

A - Appreciate those who support you and let them know
B - Be kind to others with your words and actions
C - Compliment someone sincerely
D - Donate time, money, or resources to a cause that is important to you or your whānau
E - Encourage others with positive feedback
F - Forgive someone and let go of grudges
G - Give your time to help someone in need
H - Help a neighbour or colleague
I - Inspire others with your actions
J - Join a charity event or fundraiser
K - Keep a door open for someone
L - Lend a hand to someone struggling
M - Make a meal for a friend or a neighbour
N - Notice when others could use a boost
O - Offer your skills or expertise
P - Pay it forward with a random act of kindness
Q - Quietly support someone without needing recognition
R - Reach out to offer assistance
S - Share your knowledge or tools
T - Teach someone something you know well
U - Uplift someone with a kind note or message
V - Volunteer your time for a local organisation
W - Write a thank-you note to someone
X - eXceed expectations in your generosity
Y - Your time and attention are valuable gifts
Z - Zoom in on ways to give back to your community

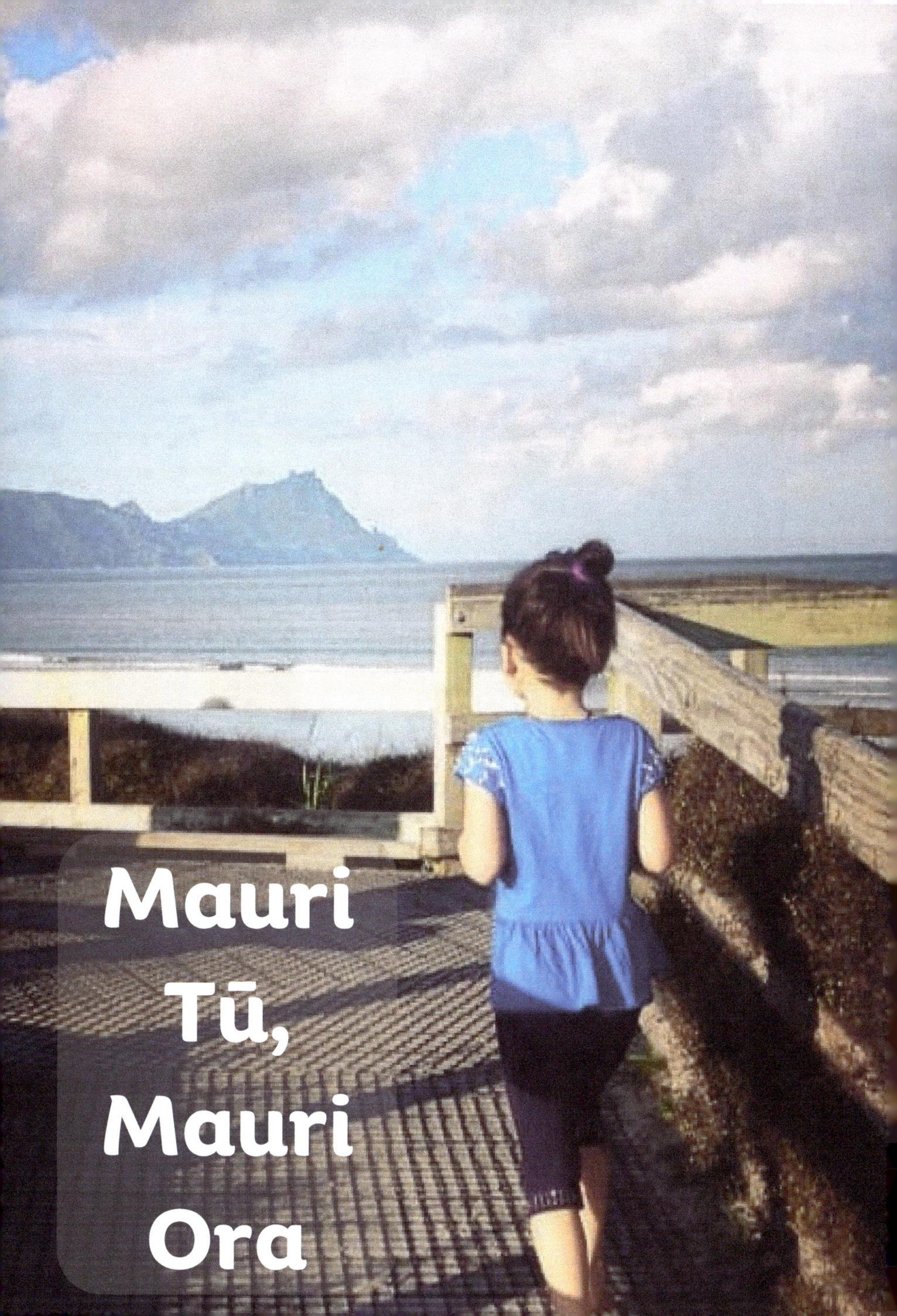

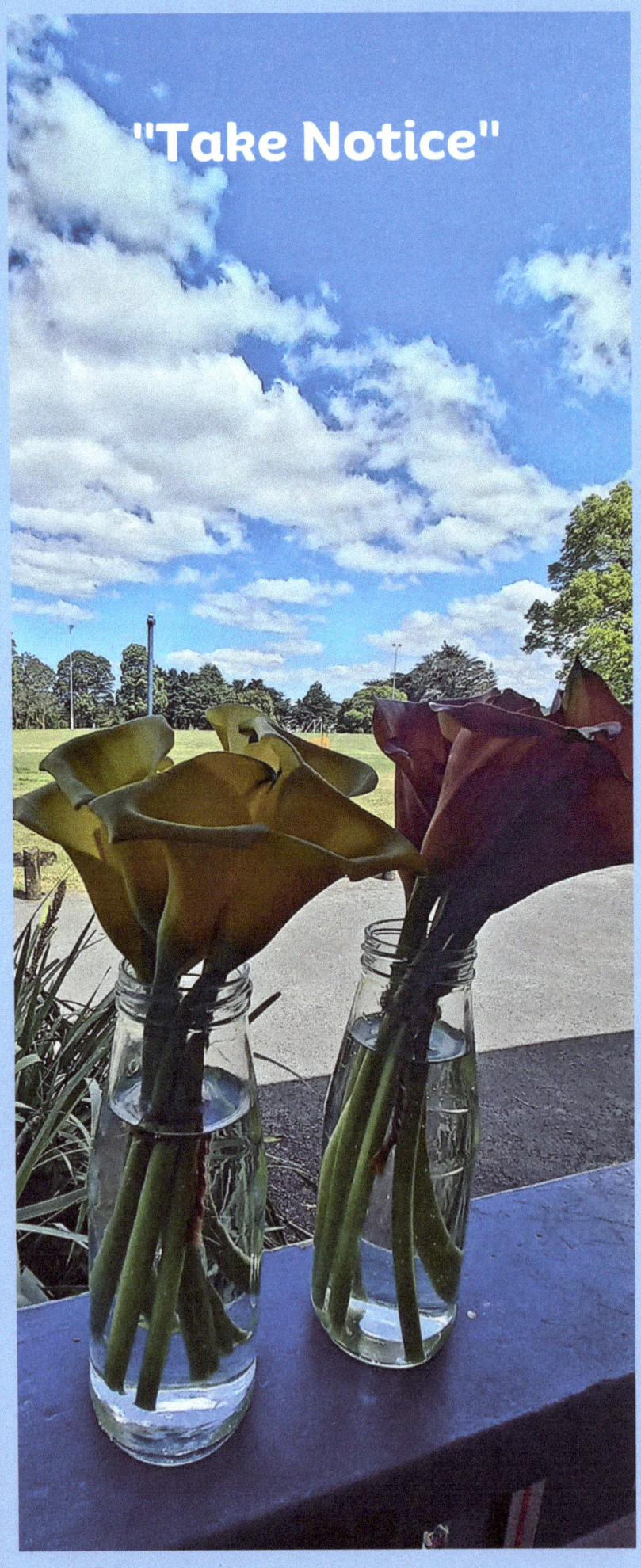

"Take Notice"

A - Ahakoa he iti he pounamu - the gift of something small, but precious
B - Breathe deeply and focus on the present
C - Celebrate your achievements, no matter how small
D - Dedicate time to reflect on your day
E - Engage your senses while eating or walking
F - Find beauty in your surroundings
G - Give attention to how you feel emotionally
H - Hear the sounds of nature around you
I - Identify things you are grateful for
J - Journal your thoughts and reflections
K - Keep a gratitude list
L - Look up at the stars or sky at night
M - Meditate for a few minutes each day
N - Notice changes in the season
O - Observe your thoughts without judgment
P - Pause to enjoy the moment
Q - Quiet your mind by focusing on your breathing
R - Reflect on what makes you happy
S - Stop and smell the flowers, literally!
T - Take time to appreciate your surroundings
U - Understand how your body feels at rest, resting is being productive
V - Visualise positive moments from your day
W - Watch and enjoy a sunset or sunrise or both, with those you love the most
X - eXperience the world with a mindful attitude
Y - Yield to moments of calm in your day
Z - Zone into the present, instead of worrying about the future

A - Ask a range of questions to deepen your understanding
B - Browse through books that interests you, create yourself a wish list
C - Challenge yourself to learn something new - a new langauge, topic of interest etc
D - Develop a new skill or hobby
E - Enroll in a course or wānanga
F - Find a mentor, role model or coach
G - Google something you've always wanted to know
H - Help someone else learn a skill you have
I - Investigate topics that pique your curiosity
J - Join a class, club, or learning community
K - Keep practicing something you've just learned - podcasts are great for that!
L - Listen to podcasts or audiobooks
M - Master a new recipe or craft
N - Nurture your love for learning
O - Open your mind to different perspectives, put your critical literacies pōtae on
P - Practice a language or musical instrument
Q - Quiz yourself on a topic of interest - this is especially fun if you do this with your whānau on Kahoot!
R - Research a topic you know little about
S - Sign up for a new challenge
T - Try a new activity like painting or coding - this can be especially fun as a whole staff
U - Utilise online tutorials or resources
V - Visit museums or cultural exhibits
W - Write about something you've learned or are passionate about
X - Xplore different cultures through learning
Y - Yearn for knowledge and new experiences, make travel plans or sit with a range of intergenerations we have a lot to learn from each other
Z - Zero in on learning opportunities in daily life

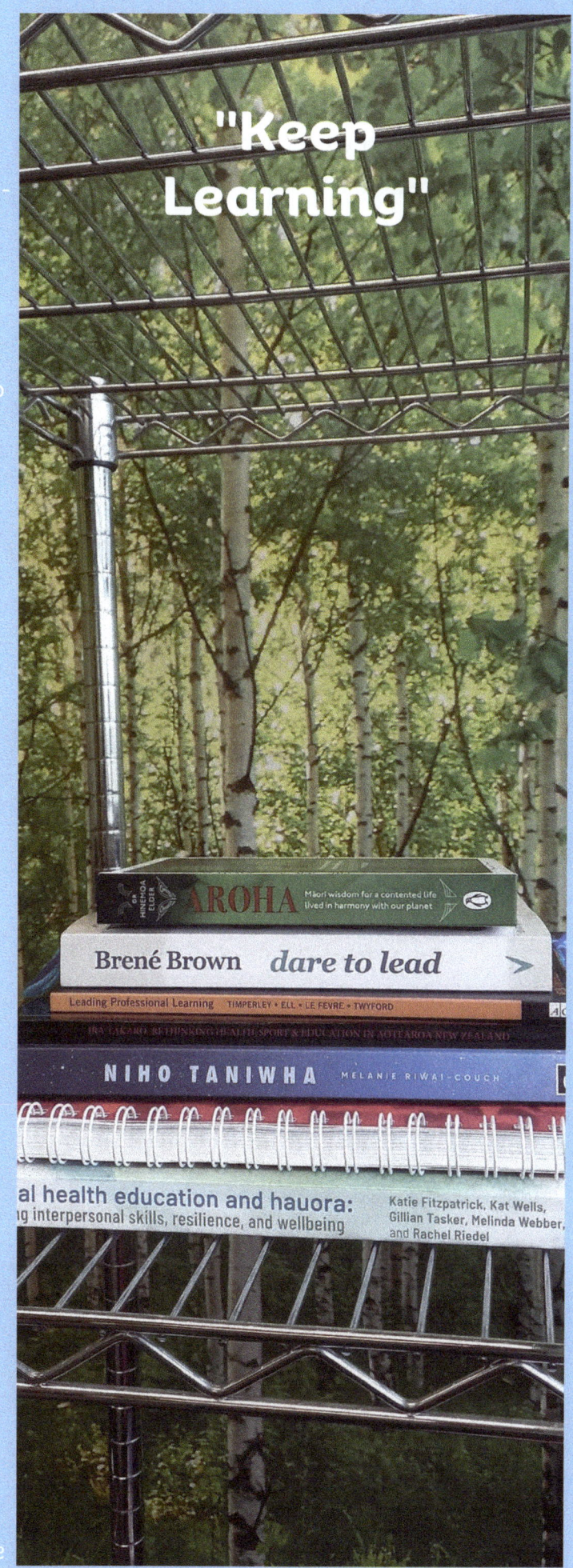

"Keep Learning"

Five Ways to Wellbeing with your Whānau

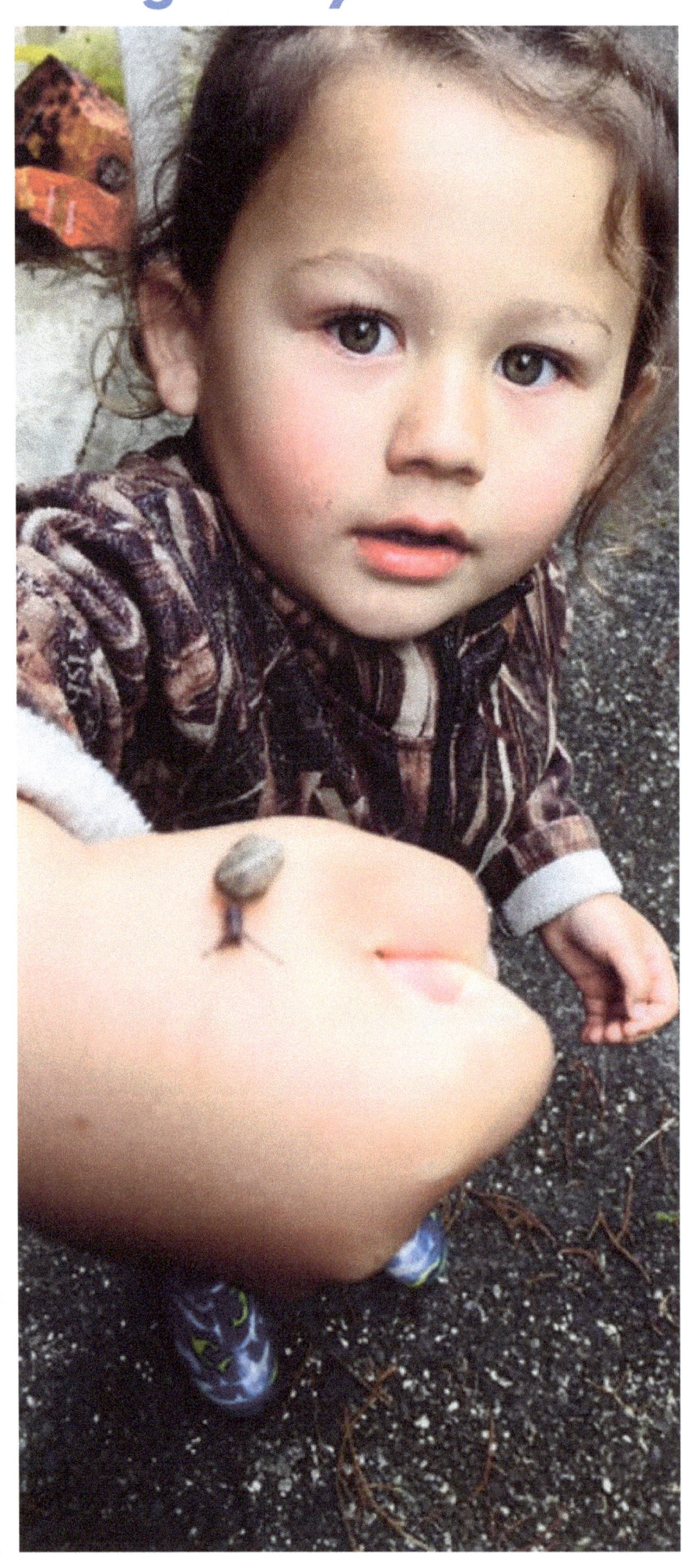

Connect: make a conscious effort today to support your whānau's emotional well-being. Check in with each whānau member and offer them your full attention, letting them know you're there for them in whatever way they need.

Be Active: support your whānau and their taha tinana by engaging in a physical activity together. Whether it's playing a sport, gardening, or dancing in the living room, being active as a family strengthens connections and promotes health.

Give: tautoko a whānau member who might need it today. Whether it's helping with chores, listening to their concerns, or spending quality time together, your support can make a big difference in their day.

Take Notice: notice the ways you can support your own well-being and that of your whānau. Maybe it's through small acts of kindness, creating a calm space at home, or simply being present. Tautoko yourself and your whānau by making hauora a priority.

Keep Learning: reflect on how you can better support your whānau's hauora. Perhaps it's learning a new recipe for a healthy meal, finding a new hobby to share, or discovering new ways to communicate and connect. Keep learning to grow together as a whānau.

Weaving Wellbeing: Connection - Movement - Growth

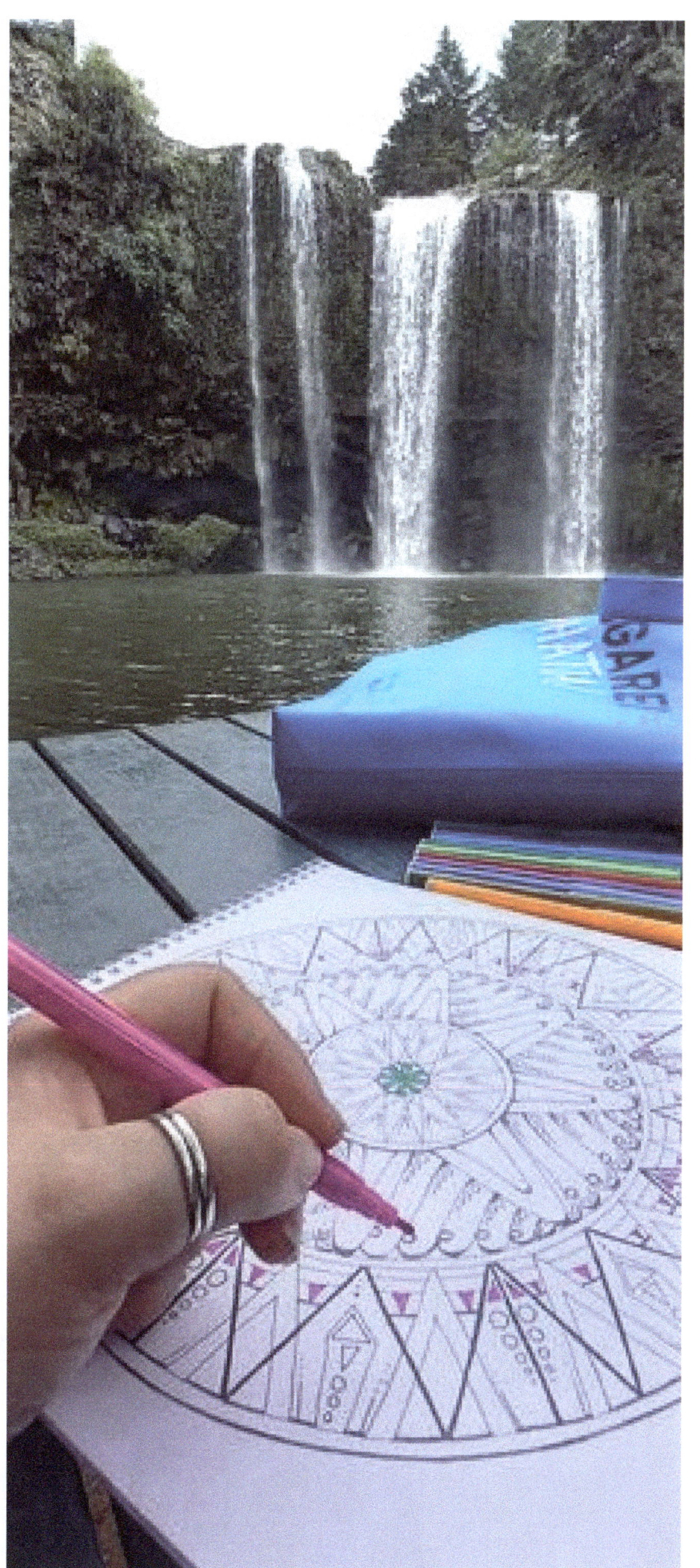

Whakawhanaunga — connect with others, whether it's a kōrero with a friend, or a simple moment of whānau togetherness. Our relationships are the harakeke that weave us into te ao.

Kia kori tinana — move in ways that feel right, stretch, run, dance, or just walk slowly. Each movement reminds you that your tinana is alive, grounded in the whenua beneath your feet.

Me aro tonu — notice what surrounds you. The birdsong in the morning, the scent of freshly fallen rain, the way the moon dances on the moana. Te taiao always has something to share, if you pause to listen.

Ako tonu — keep learning, whether it's a new skill, a story of our tīpuna, or a different way of seeing the world. Your hinengaro expands, as you explore the unknown, growing with each discovery.

Aroha atu, aroha mai — give with kindness, not just material things, your time, your manaakitanga. In giving, you nurture both others and yourself and the wairua of generosity flows through us all.

Erin Steel 2024

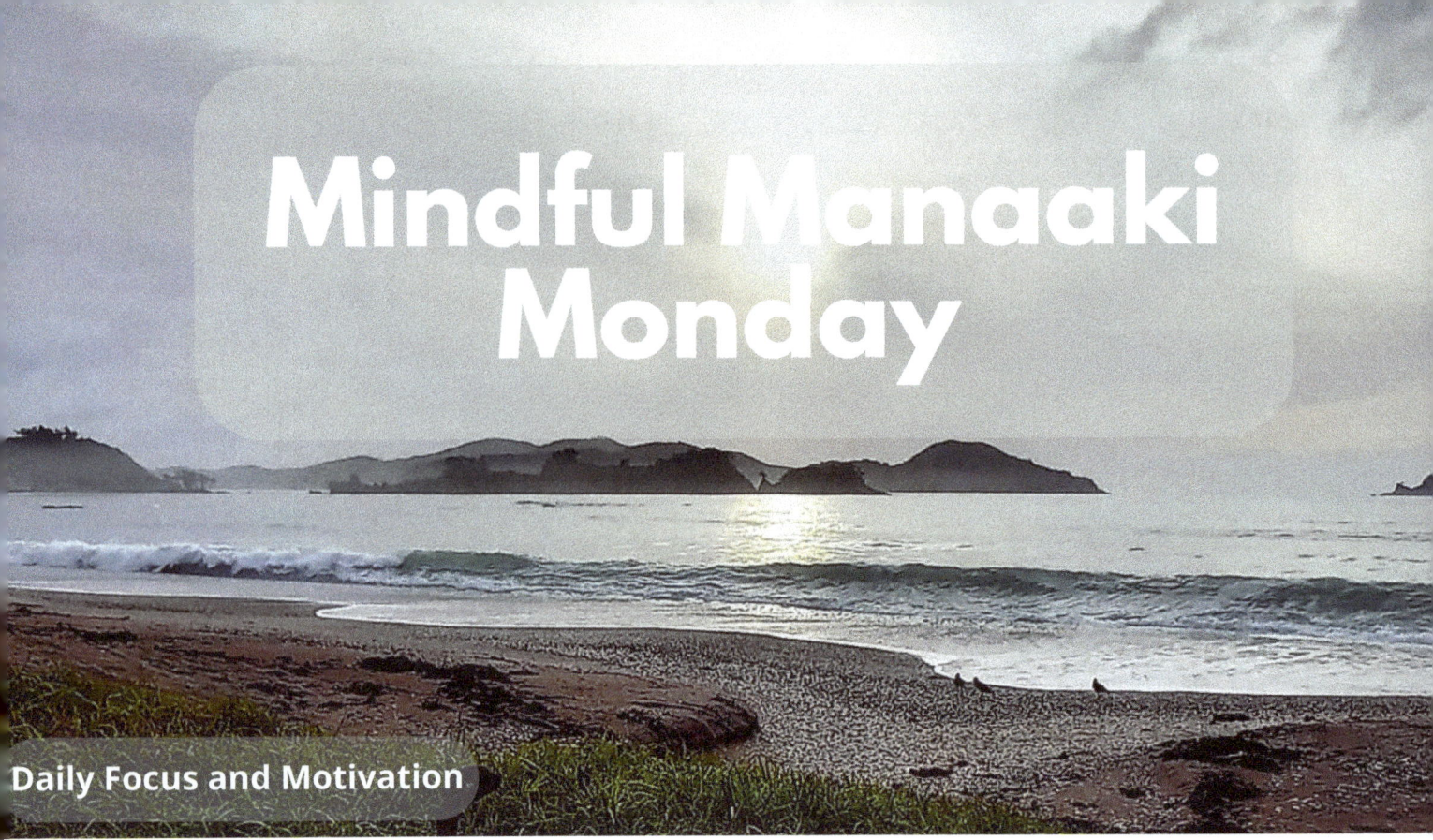

Mindful Manaaki Monday

Daily Focus and Motivation

Magical meditation: setting your daily / weekly intentions
- Spend 10 minutes meditating. Use this time to set clear intentions for the day. Focus on one key intention that aligns with your vision and goals.

Manaaki moments: acts of kindness
- Perform a small act of kindness for someone. It could be a compliment, a thank you note, or helping out a colleague or friend.

Magical mandalas: creative pause
- Take 15 minutes to color or create a mandala. Allow your mind to relax and focus on the patterns and colors, enhancing your mindfulness.

Mindful Meal: healthy treat
- Prepare a nutritious and delicious snack or meal. While eating, practice mindful eating by savouring each bite and appreciating the flavors.

Motivated Planning: Review Goals
- Spend some time reviewing your goals and progress. Adjust your action plan as needed and celebrate any achievements.

Morning magic: vision board vibes
- Start your day by revisiting your goals, dreams and aspirations with your vision board. Reflect on how you'll achieve it and why it's important.

Mindful movement: quick walk & talk
- Take a 10-minute walk, whether it's around your neighborhood or through a nearby park. Use this time to focus on your breath and be present in the moment.

Motivated moves: energising activity
- Engage in a quick physical activity that boosts your energy. It could be a short workout, a dance break, or some stretching exercises.

Magical evening: relax & reflect
- End your day with a relaxing activity that brings you joy, like reading, journaling, or listening to calming music. Reflect on your day and how you've embraced the themes of motivation, magic, mindfulness, and manaaki.

Tautoko Tuesday

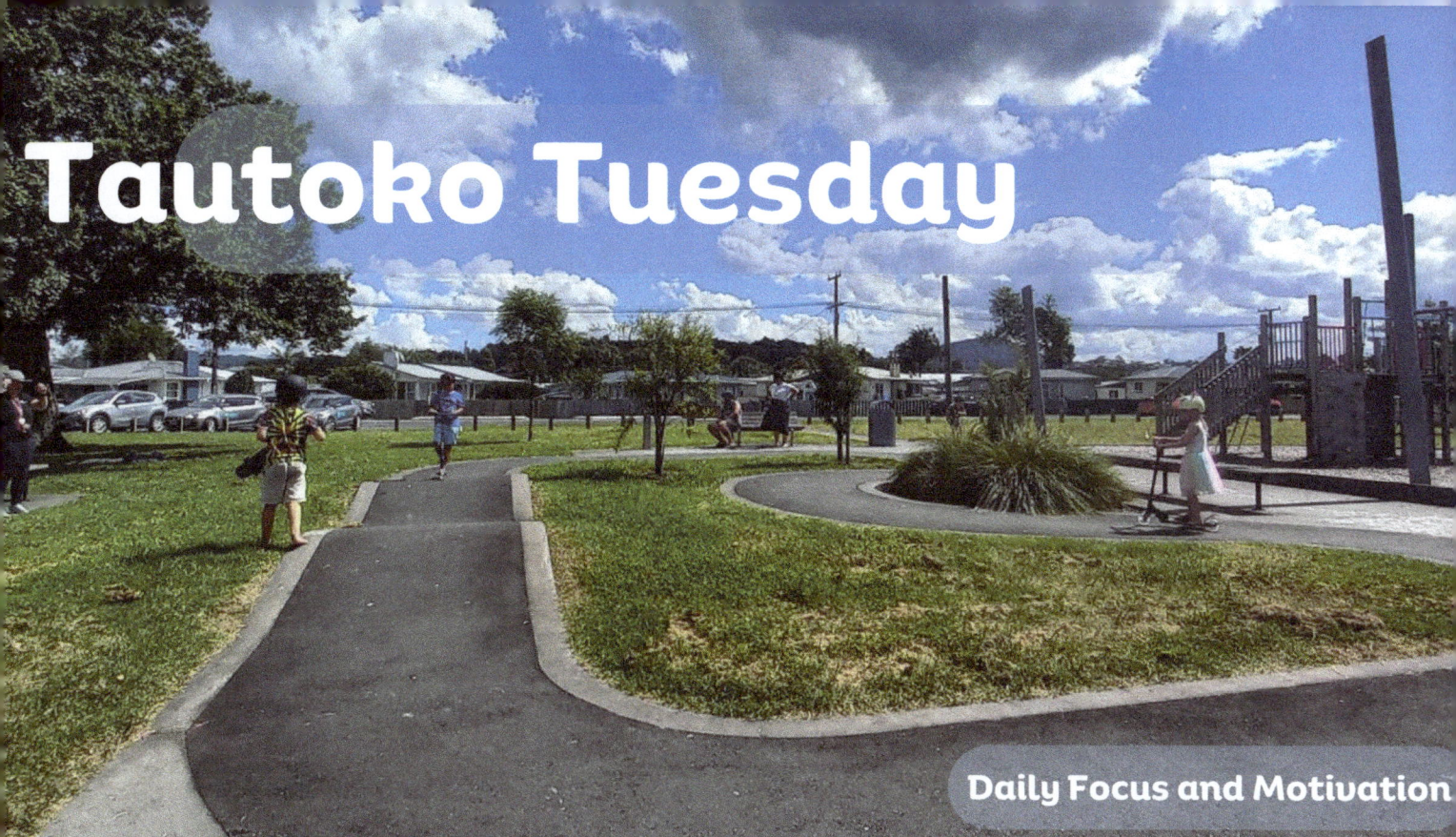

Daily Focus and Motivation

Connect:
Reach out to a colleague today with words of encouragement or an offer of help. Your support can make a big difference in their day and reinforce the sense of community within your school.

Be Active:
Support a colleague by inviting them to join you for a physical activity, like a walk or a quick game outside. Being active together can boost your well-being and strengthen your connection. How many other opportunities are there to engage with each other?

Keep Learning:
Reflect on the ways you can offer more tautoko in your daily life. Consider learning about new ways to support your colleagues and students, enhancing the collective well-being of your whānau, school and community.

Give:
Tautoko your team by sharing a resource, tip, or strategy that has worked well for you. Giving knowledge and support can help others feel more confident and capable.

Take Notice:
Pay attention to how your colleagues are doing today. If you notice someone who seems stressed or overwhelmed, offer your tautoko through a kind word or gesture of support.

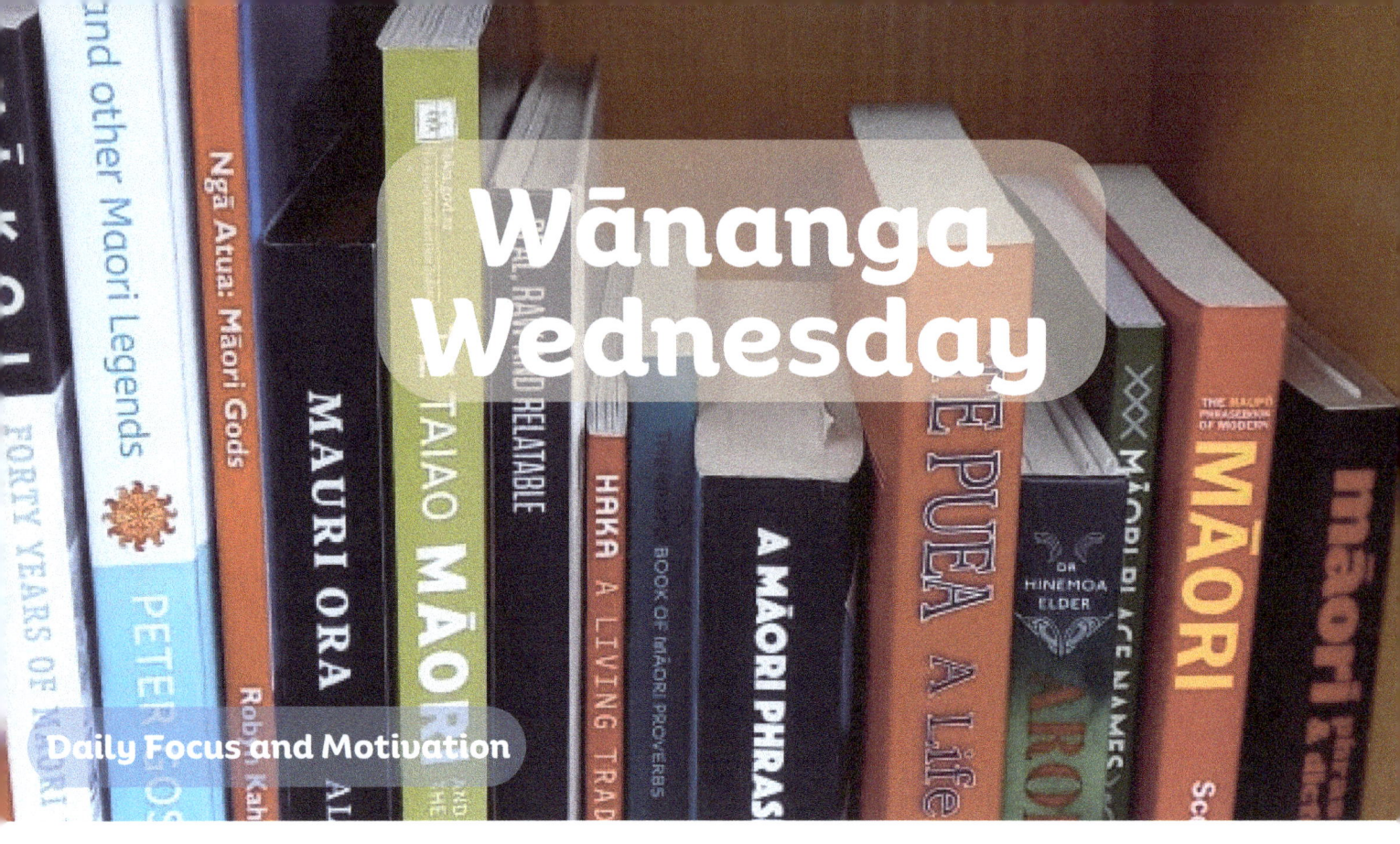

Wānanga Wednesday

Daily Focus and Motivation

Strong relationships with others are an essential part of building resilience and boosting wellbeing. They set us up well for when life is tough. Mental Health Foundation of NZ

Me Whakawhanaunga - Connect this week, carve out time for a whānau wānanga where everyone shares one highlight and one challenge from their week. How does this open kōrero strengthen your connections and enhance the well-being of each whānau member?

Me Kori Tonu - Be Active plan an active whānau adventure—whether it's a hike in the ngahere, an afternoon at the beach, or a family sports game. Reflect on how being physically active together enhances your well-being and recharges your energy for the week ahead.

Me Aro Tonu - Take Notice at your next whānau kai or gathering, take a moment to fully appreciate the presence of each family member. Notice how being truly present with your whānau uplifts your mood and well-being.

Me Ako Tonu - Keep Learning organise a whānau learning experience, such as trying out a new recipe together, learning a new game, or exploring a cultural tradition. How does engaging in this learning together enhance your well-being and foster a sense of growth?

Tukua - Give encourage each whānau member to perform a small act of kindness this week, whether it's helping with a task, offering a kind word, or spending time with someone who needs support. Reflect on how these acts of giving back to your whānau enrich your well-being and strengthen your connections.

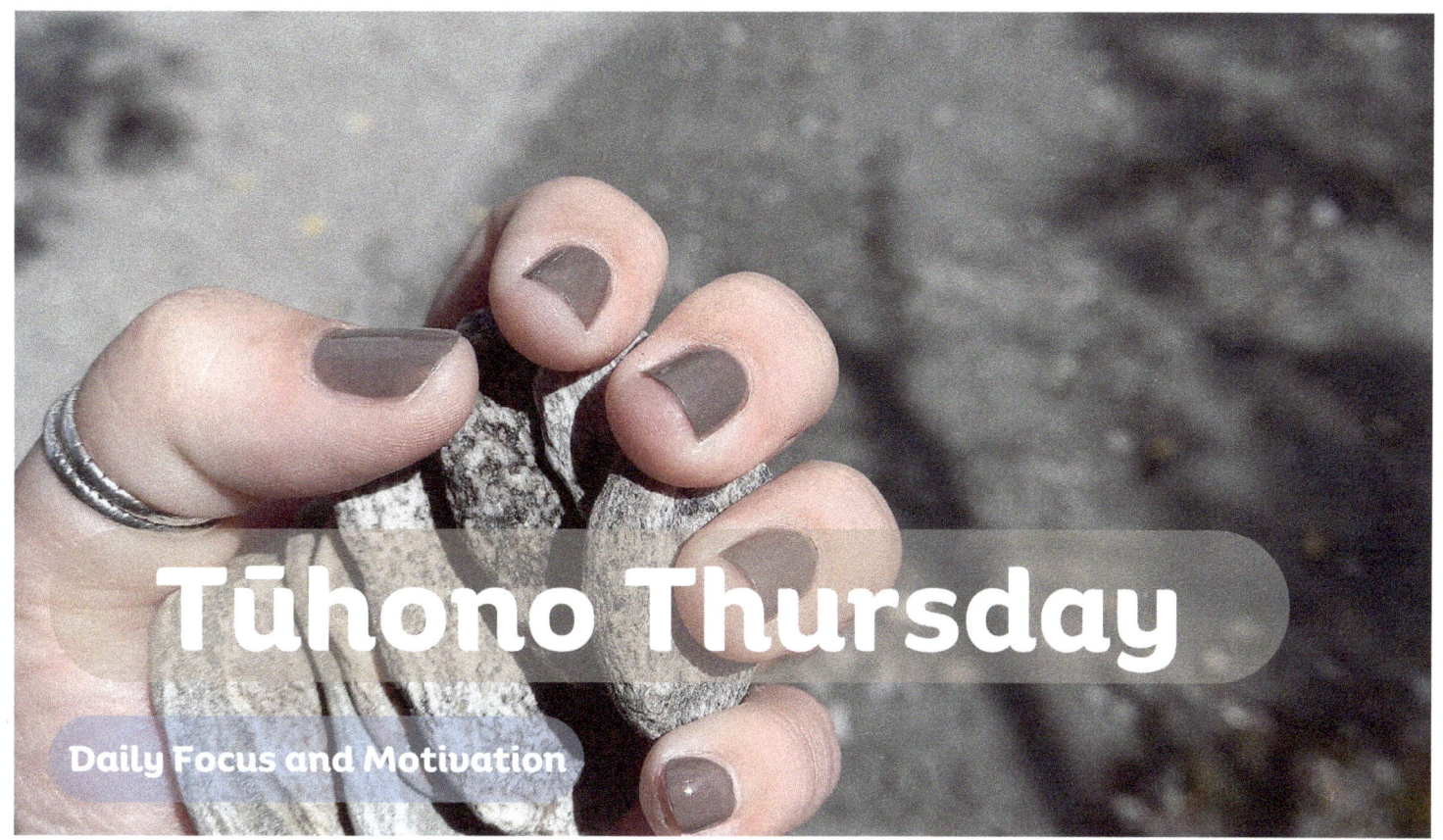

Tūhono Thursday
Daily Focus and Motivation

I miss the good old days where everyone knew their neighbours. Let's bring that back - I know I am proud to be part of our community!

I used to think it was random when my mum used to do these things when I was a young person, now I understand why and the value this can have 😊

- Kia Ora koutou katoa, Ko Erin Steel toku ingoa. Ko wai au? Ko wai to ingoa? No hea koe? Are all intros and pātai that you could use when you introduce yourself.
- Have you had a new neighbour move in - why not introduce yourself and offer a warm welcome.
- Strike up a conversation with another parent you haven't connected with before.
- Say "Kia Ora" to a neighbour you see on your morning walk and introduce yourself.
- If you've been out hunting or gathering or have some spare kai - fish, tuatua, etc... share it with your neighbours 😊 (this one's my fav)
- Knock on the door of a neighbour you haven't met and introduce yourself.
- Ask a neighbour about local activities or community events to get involved.
- Organise a neighbourhood potluck or gathering to meet more people in your community. (Even better, if you live on a quiet street, ask me how you could organise a neighbourhood play street - intergenerational play is beneficial for everyone of all ages!)
- Join a local community garden or volunteer group and introduce yourself to fellow members.
- Offer to help a neighbour with yard work or a home project to break the ice.
- Host a casual game night or barbecue and invite neighbours you haven't met yet.
- Attend a local town hall or community meeting to introduce yourself and get involved.
- Bring a small gift or baked goods to a new neighbour as a welcoming gesture.
- Participate in or organise a community cleanup event and use the opportunity to meet others.
- Organise a Play Street on a regular basis.
- Attend a local workshop, art class, or fitness class and introduce yourself to fellow participants.

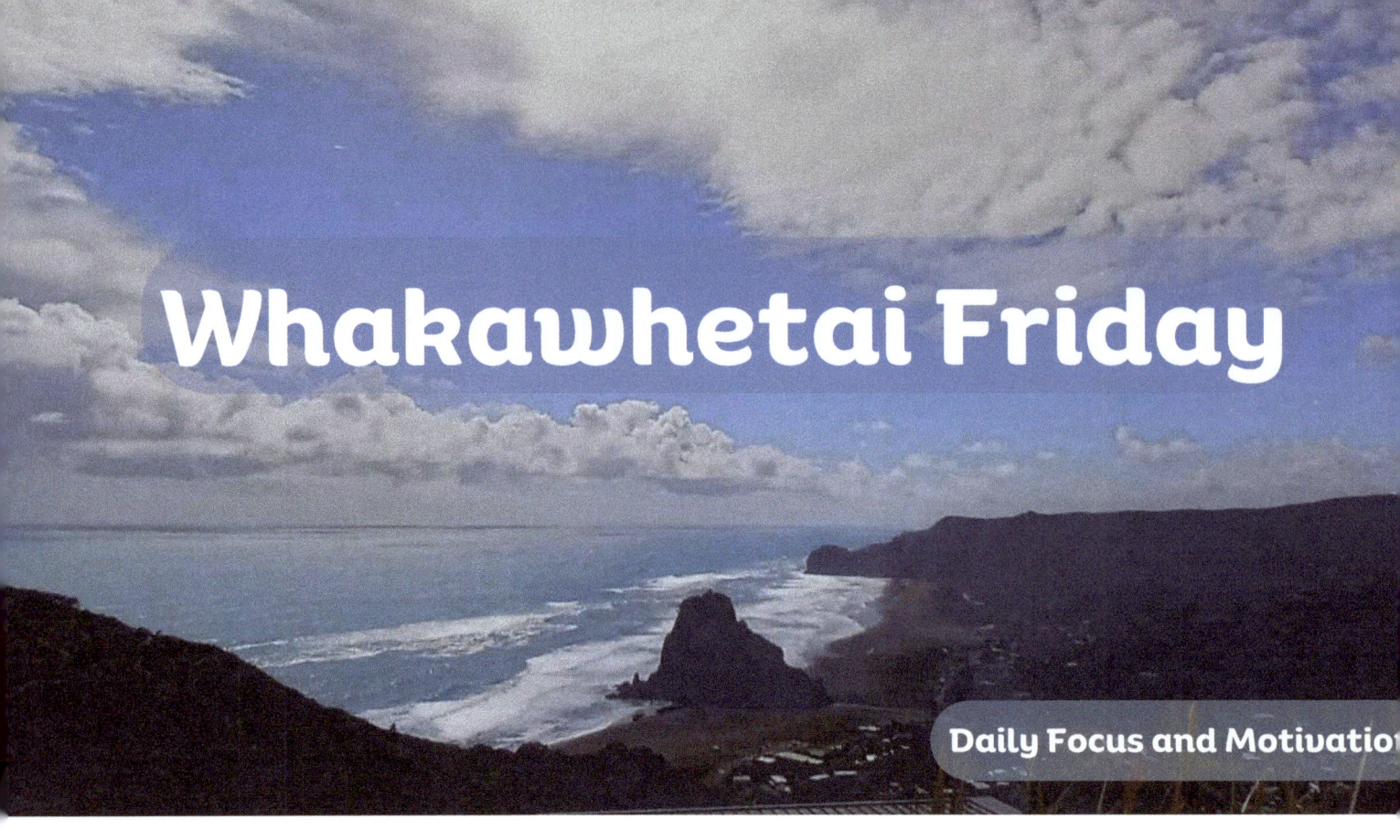

Whakawhetai Friday

Daily Focus and Motivation

Continuing with the whānau theme. Too often our whānau get the leftovers of whatever energies we have left. How might you prioritise you and your whānau today or this week?

Me Whakawhanaunga - Connect
- Hold a whānau meeting outside to kōrero about aspirations, nature and well-being.
- Spend time in the outdoors, taking turns capturing pictures of the taiao and sharing stories behind each photo.
- Play classic games like hide and seek, tag, or charades in the backyard or park to connect and have fun together.

Tukua - Give
- Join a beach, park, or river clean-up to give back to the environment as a whānau.
- Plant and nurture a māra kai at home, giving back to the earth while growing vegetables, herbs, or native plants.
- Create bird feeders using recycled materials and hang them outside to attract native manu, providing them with nourishment.

Me Aro Tonu - Take Notice
- Take a quiet walk, focusing on the sounds, smells, and sights of nature. Afterwards, discuss what everyone noticed.
- Bring notebooks and art supplies outside to draw, write, or paint about what you see, hear, and feel in the taiao.
- Gather early in the morning or late in the evening to watch the sunrise or sunset, taking notice of the changing colours and light.

Me Ako Tonu - Keep Learning
- Research and identify native plants in your area, discussing their uses and significance in te ao Māori.
- Create a "bug hotel" using natural materials to learn about local insects and their role in the ecosystem.
- Head outside on a clear night to observe the stars and learn more.

Me Kori Tonu - Be Active
- Choose a local track, maunga, or ngahere to explore together, getting exercise while enjoying the beauty of nature.
- Set up an obstacle course using natural materials like sticks, stones and ropes for a fun, active challenge.
- Take a portable speaker outside, play some waiata and have a dance party in nature to move your tinana joyfully.

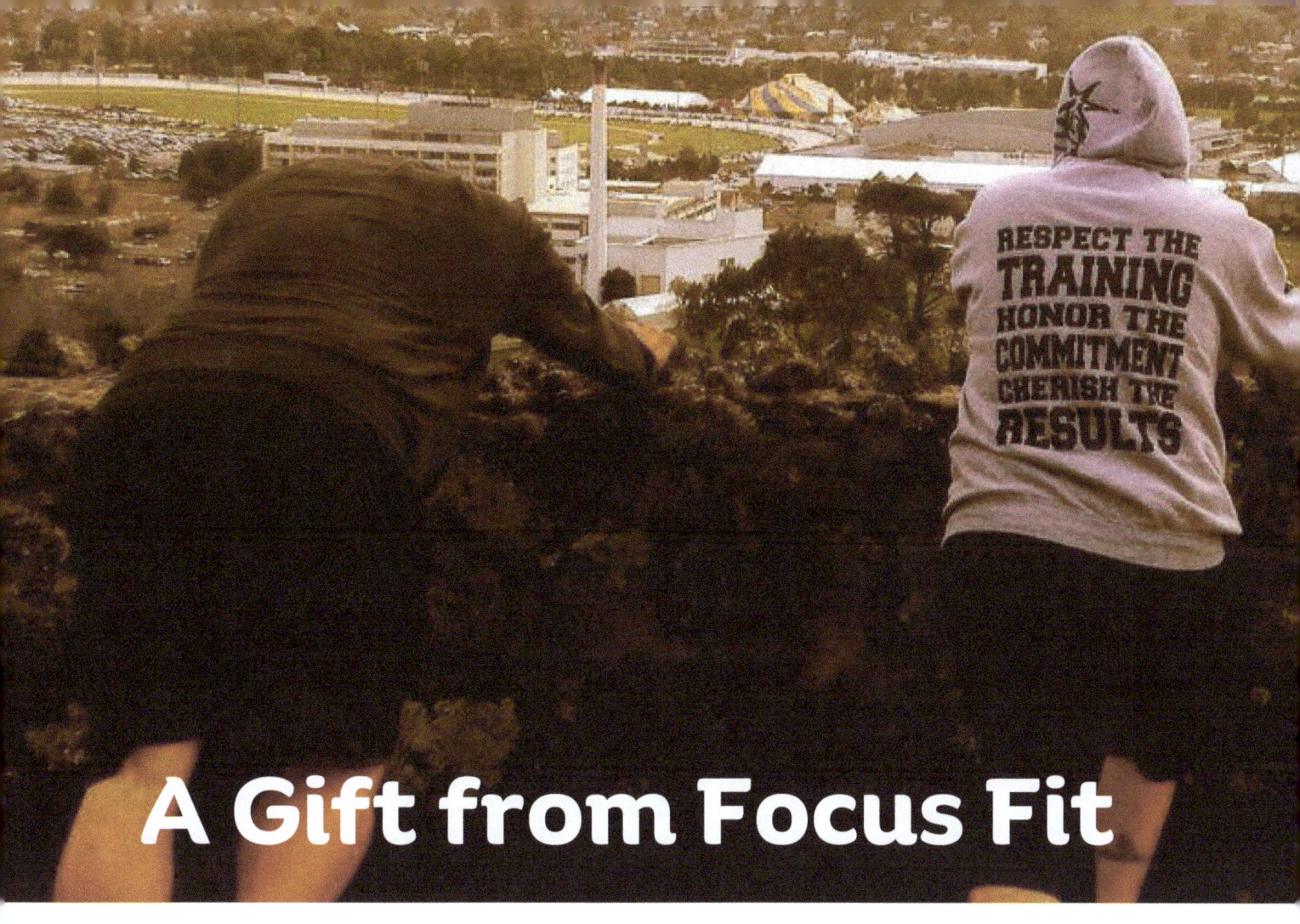

A Gift from Focus Fit

Start with what matters,
the big rocks, clear and steady,
held in your hands before the rush of distractions sweeps them aside.

Work in bursts—focused, sharp,
a rhythm of effort and rest,
like breathing in, like tides,
a balance of giving and gathering back.

Take time to move — step away, stretch, let your body remind you that energy flows when we do.

Pause to look back, a quiet review of what you've built this week, this month, this year, this decade…

Successes stand tall,
lessons ripple underneath,
guiding you forward.

And as the week closes,
set space for yourself. Find your joy, your stillness,
something just for you.

Let it be the bridge
that carries you into the weekend, refreshed, ready,
with time well spent.

Erin Steel 2014

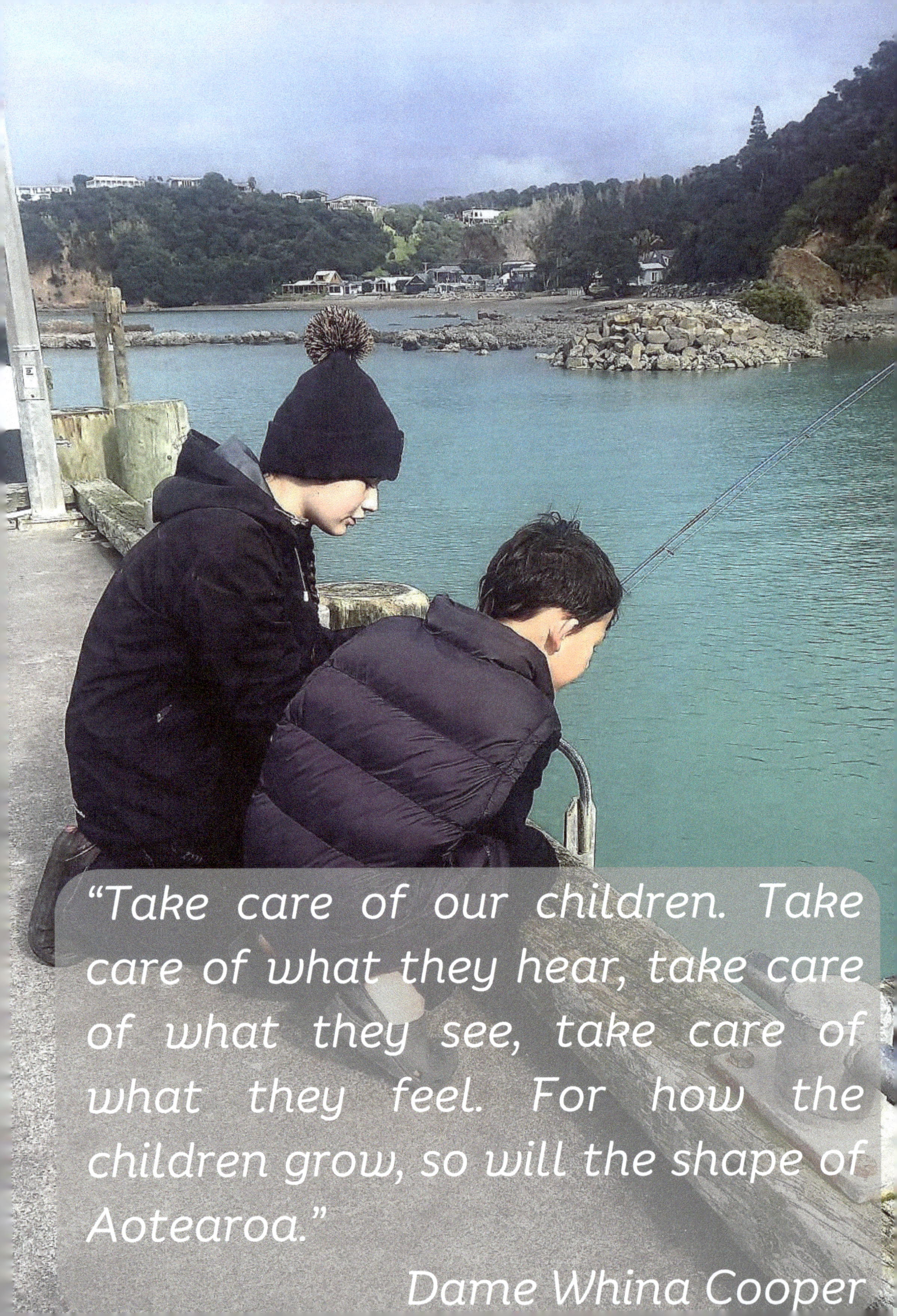

"Take care of our children. Take care of what they hear, take care of what they see, take care of what they feel. For how the children grow, so will the shape of Aotearoa."

Dame Whina Cooper

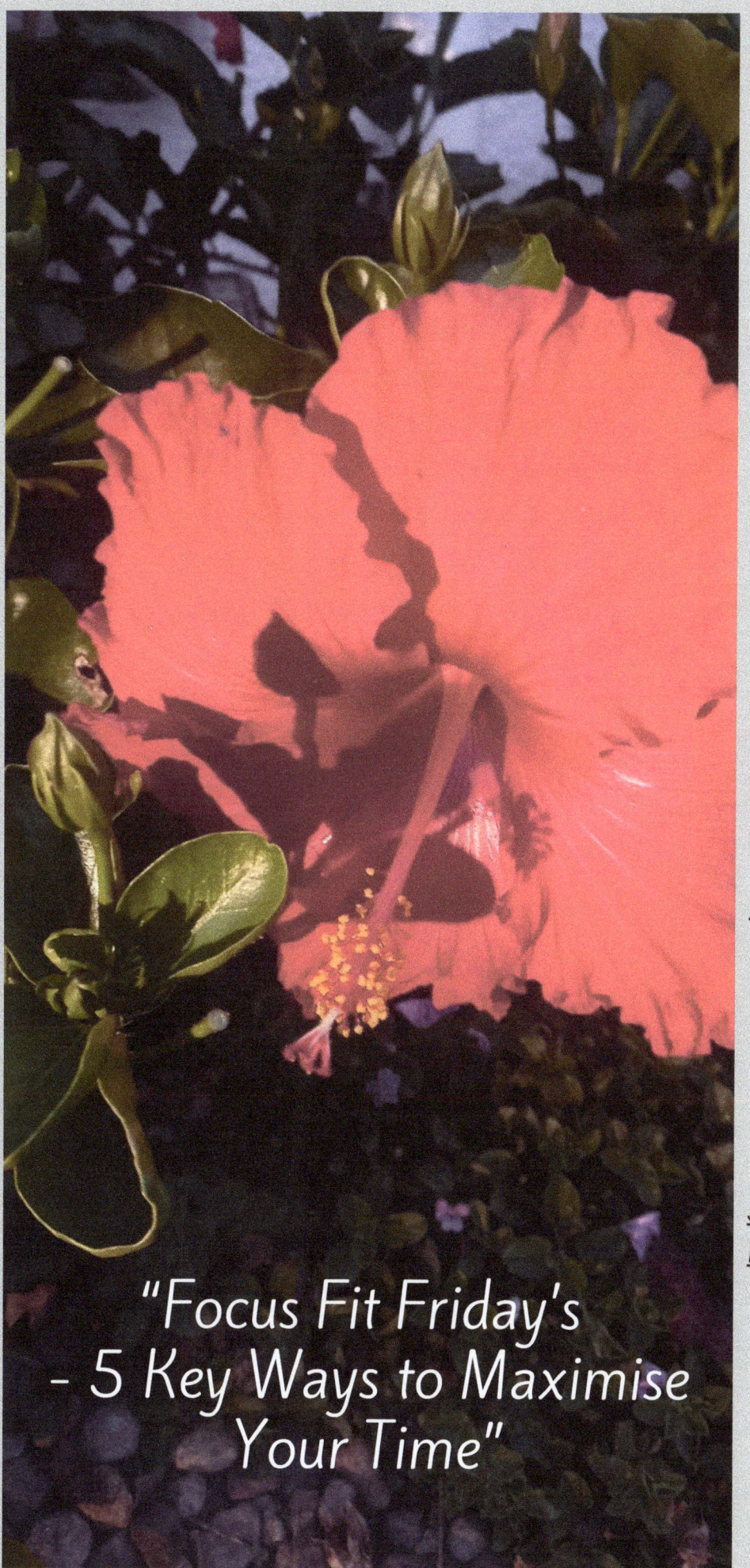

"Focus Fit Friday's - 5 Key Ways to Maximise Your Time"

<u>Prioritise what matters (Big Rocks First)</u>:
- Identify top 3 priorities for the day.
- Set aside 15-30 minutes in the morning to organise and focus on key tasks.

<u>Use short, focused work bursts</u>:
- Implement time-blocking (e.g., Pomodoro method).
- Work for 25-30 minutes, followed by a 5-minute break.

<u>Incorporate active breaks</u>:
- Schedule 10-15 minute movement breaks every hour.
- Use the time to walk, stretch, or do a quick workout.

<u>Review, reflect and plan ahead</u>:
- Spend 15-20 minutes reviewing the week's successes and lessons.
- Plan your first task for Monday to start the next week strong.

<u>Set intentional time for well-being</u>:
- Block out an hour at the end of Friday for self-care or a fun activity.
- Use this time to recharge and transition into the weekend.

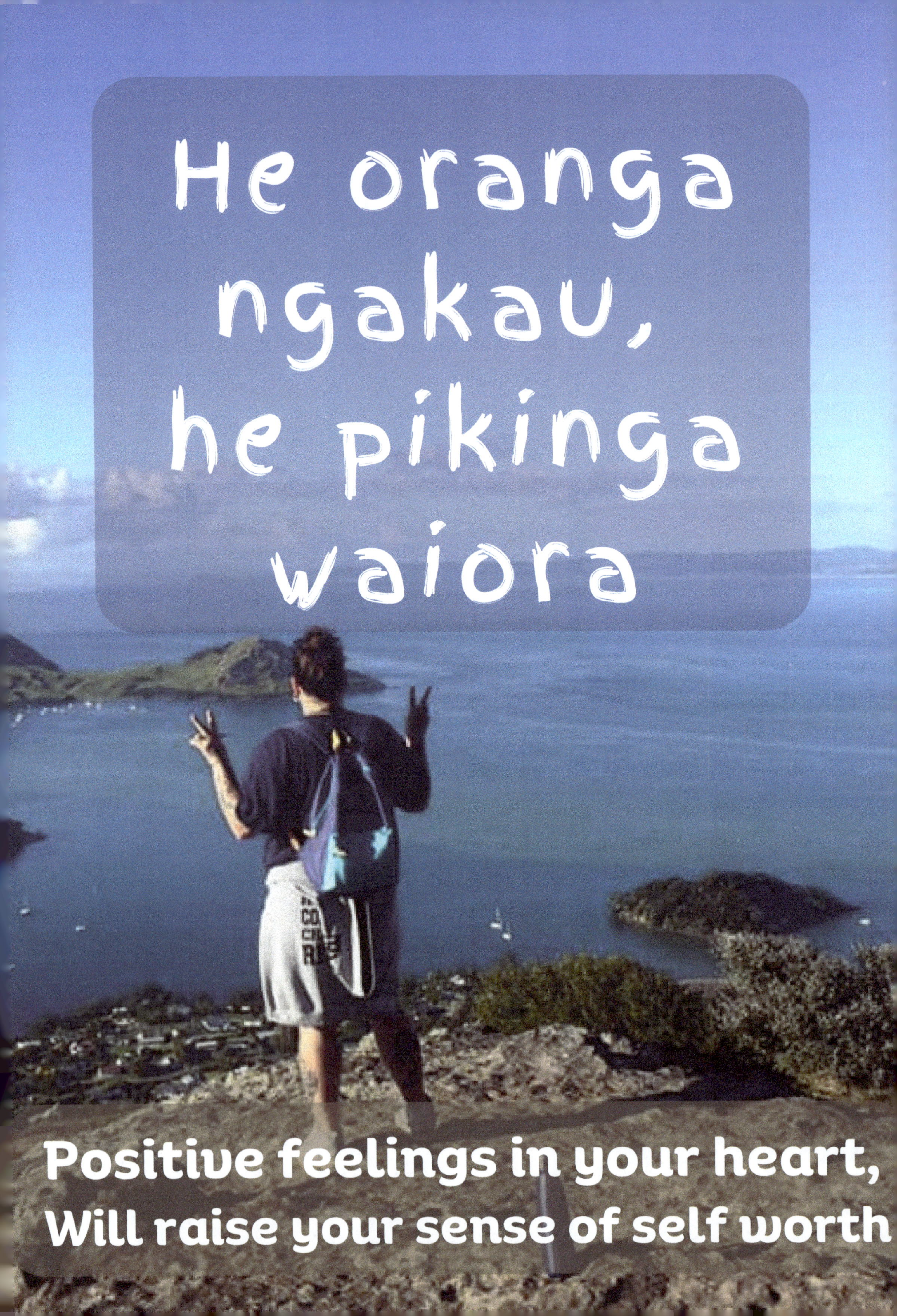

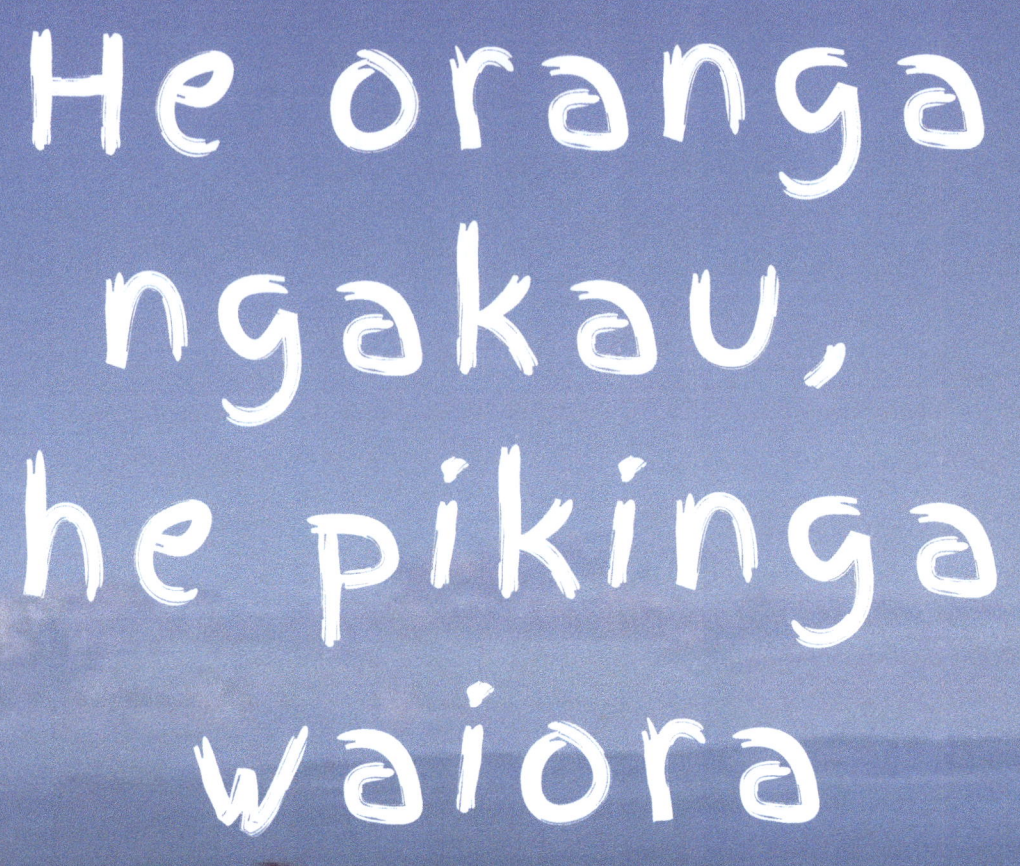

He oranga ngakau, he pikinga waiora

Positive feelings in your heart, Will raise your sense of self worth

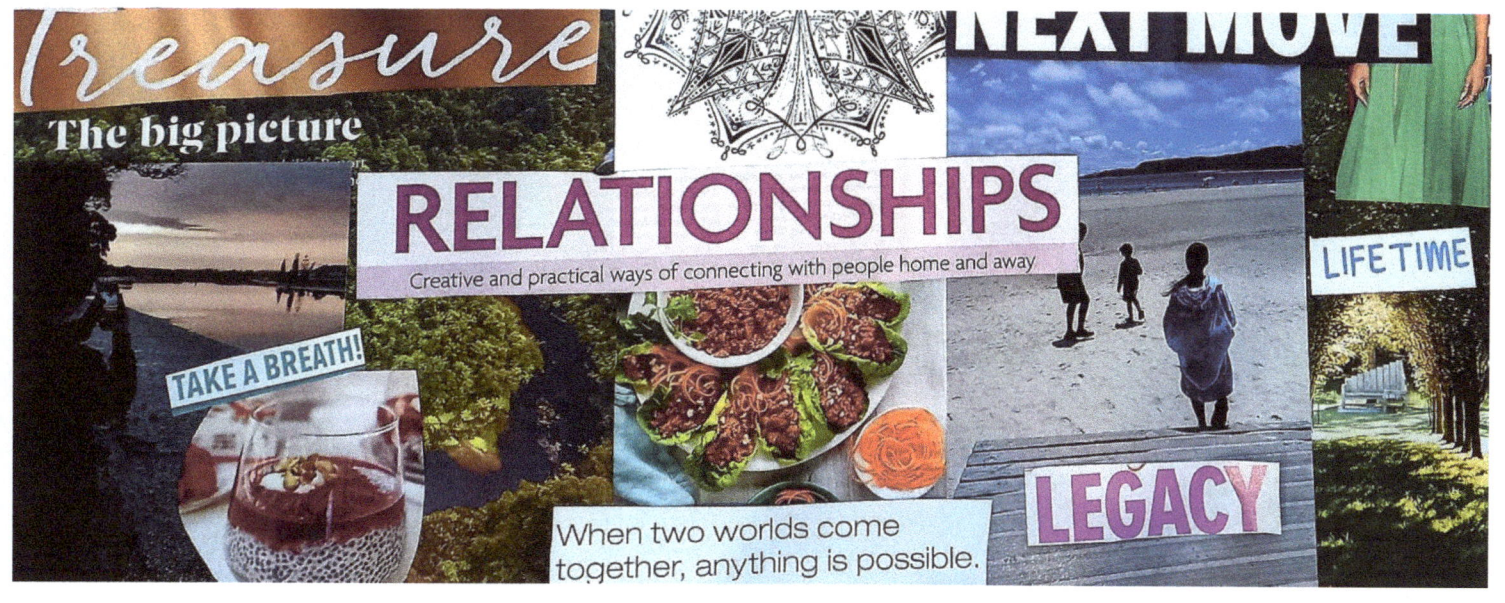

Mindfulness Month
Encouragement for kaiako facing mental health challenges

These are just a few of the important lessons I've learned from colleagues and professionals over the years and along the way (especially post concussion):

Seek professional help early
Please know, it's okay to ask for help. Reach out to a mental health professional like a counsellor or therapist when things feel overwhelming. Early intervention can make a big difference. The Mental Health Foundation of NZ has a directory of services to help you find the right support.

Build your support network
As a community of kaiako, you can find trusted colleagues, friends and whānau to connect with and who will listen and support you. Having a safe space to share your thoughts and feelings can lighten the load.
Consider peer support groups, where you can talk with other kaiako facing similar challenges.

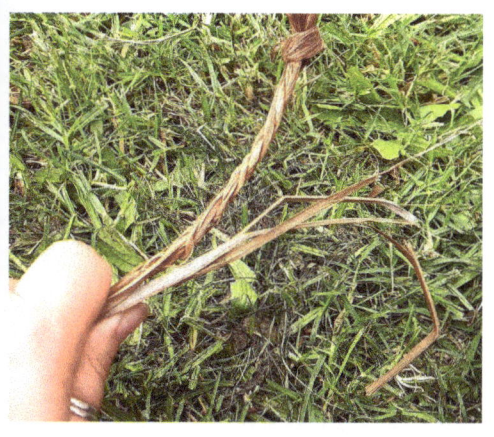

Practice self-compassion
On those really challenging days, it takes a lot of energy to do even the little things. Be kind to yourself. You're doing the best you can in a demanding role. Give yourself permission to take breaks and practice self-care without guilt.

Use the 5 Ways to Wellbeing

Incorporate 'brain breaks' throughout the day to avoid burnout—take a quick walk, listen to calming music, or enjoy something that brings you joy and makes you smile.

Set healthy boundaries
Something I often share when working with kaiako is, it's ok to say "no". Prioritising ourselves by saying "no", we are saying our workload is a bit much at the moment, I need time to breathe and manage my current mahi. It's important to establish clear boundaries between mahi and personal time to protect your mental health. Work/Life satisfaction comes to mind.

Take small, manageable steps
Don't feel pressure to fix everything at once. Break tasks down into small steps, focusing on one thing at a time. Celebrate each little accomplishment—progress is progress.

Remember you're not alone
Many kaiako face similar challenges and it's important to know that you're part of a wider community that supports and understands you. Reach out to your network, professional groups, or local mental health services for additional resources.

Focus on what you can control
Easier said than done I know... Let's focus on what's within our control and let go of things that aren't. We can shift our energy towards positive actions that we can take and remind ourselves that we're doing our best in a challenging role.

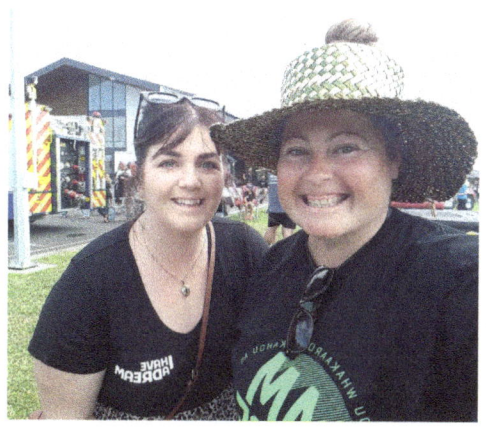

Building a strong support system, utilising tools from the Mental Health Foundation and leaning into strategies like the 5 Ways to Wellbeing, we can strengthen our mental health and well-being as a kaiako. Your mahi is important and so are you!

Food for Thought

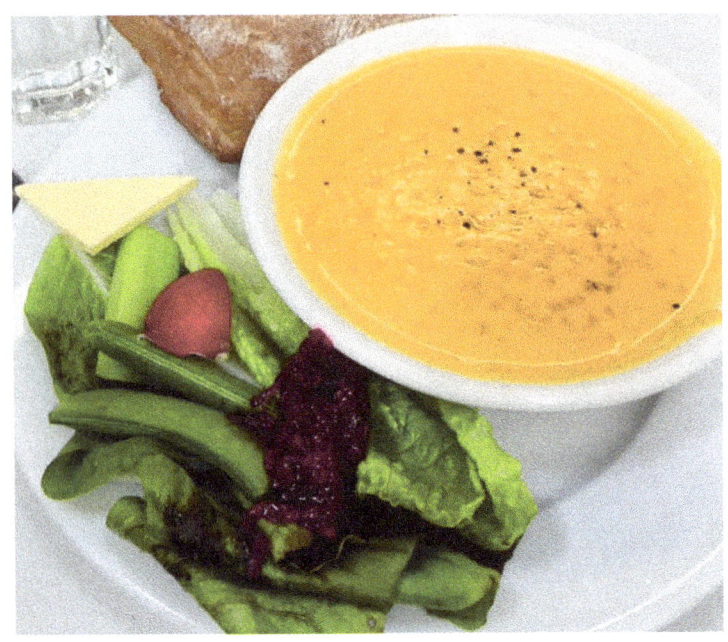

Have you ever stopped to think about the fuel we give our minds and bodies? Just like the quality of food impacts our physical health, the thoughts we consume shape our well-being. What we focus on and feed our minds with—whether it's positivity, learning, or stress—can uplift us or weigh us down.

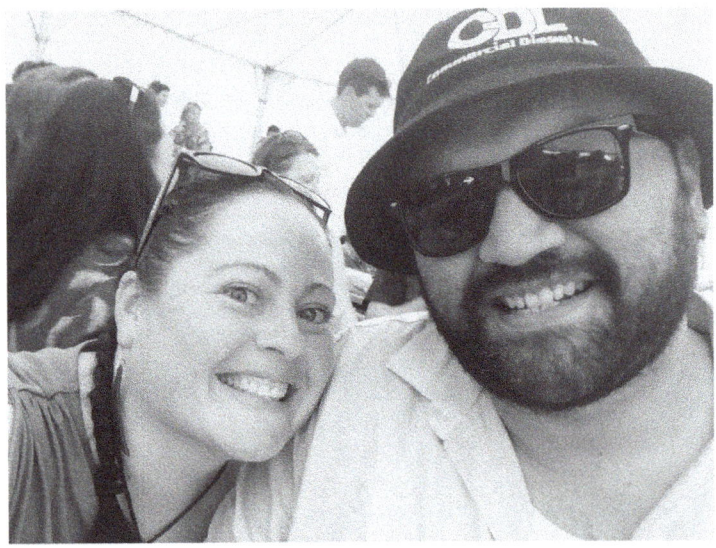

Take a moment today to nourish both body and mind: Eat mindfully. Notice how the food you choose energises or affects your mood.

Feed your mind. What are you reading, listening to, or thinking about? Is it inspiring growth or holding you back? Balance. Just as with food, it's all about balance—indulge in things that bring you joy and make sure you're fueling yourself with what helps you thrive.

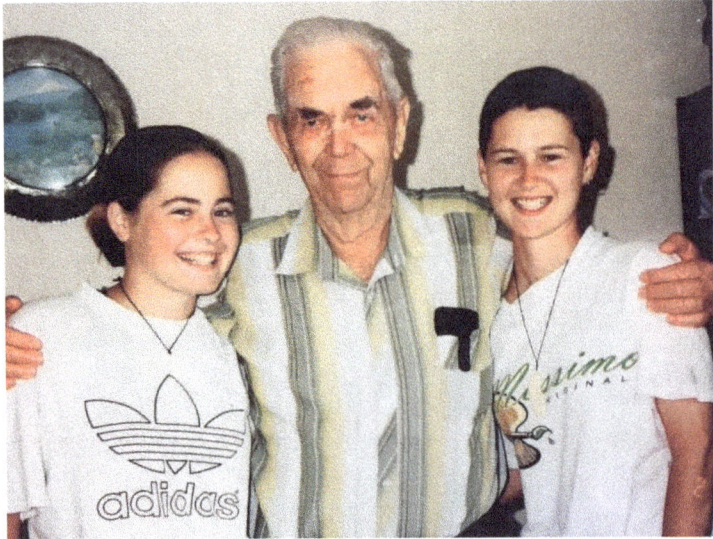

What's one thing you can do today to fuel your well-being from the inside out? 🌱

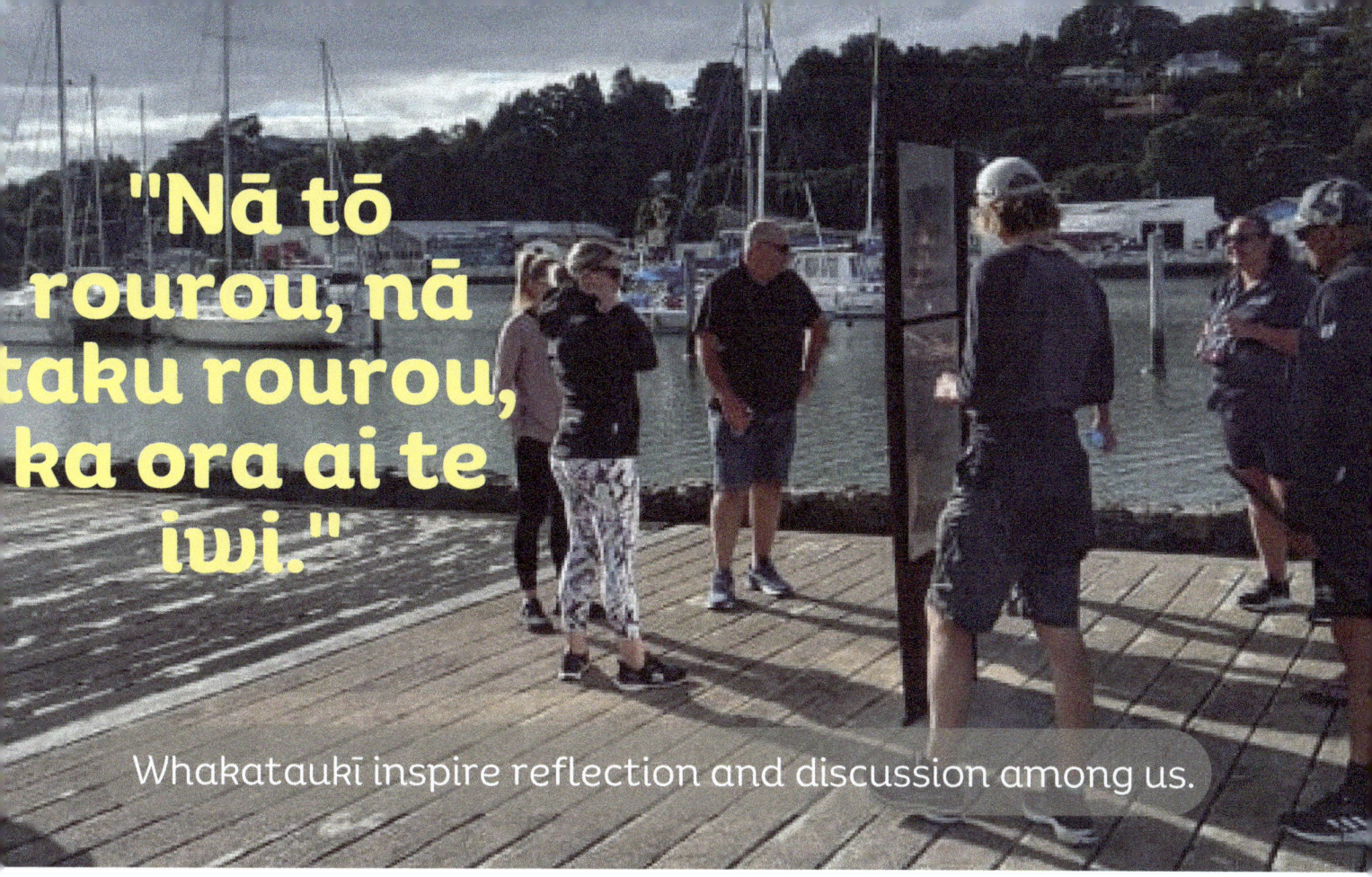

Whakataukī inspire reflection and discussion among us.

"He iti hau marangai, e tū te pāhokahoka."
(A little storm and then a rainbow appears.)
Perseverance and resilience
Prompt: Reflect on a challenge you've faced this week. How did you find your rainbow at the end of it?

Togetherness and whanaungatanga
"Nā tō rourou, nā taku rourou, ka ora ai te iwi."
(With your food basket and my food basket, the people will thrive.)
Prompt: Share a time this week when collaboration made a difference in your work or life. How does working together enhance our collective hauora?

"Ko te kai a te rangatira he kōrero."
(The food of chiefs is dialogue.)
Leadership and growth
Prompt: Discuss how effective communication has played a role in your leadership journey. How can we use kōrero to uplift and support each other?

"Ko te manu e kai ana i te miro, nōna te ngahere. Ko te manu e kai ana i te mātauranga, nōna te ao."
(The bird that feasts on the miro berry belongs to the forest. The bird that feasts on knowledge belongs to the world.)
Learning and knowledge
Prompt: Reflect on something new you learned this week. How does acquiring knowledge expand your horizons and opportunities?

"Whāia te iti kahurangi, ki te tūohu koe me he maunga teitei."
(Seek the treasure you value most dearly, if you bow your head, let it be to a lofty mountain.)
Determination and courage
Prompt: Identify a goal or aspiration you are currently pursuing. What steps are you taking to reach it and how do you stay motivated when faced with obstacles?

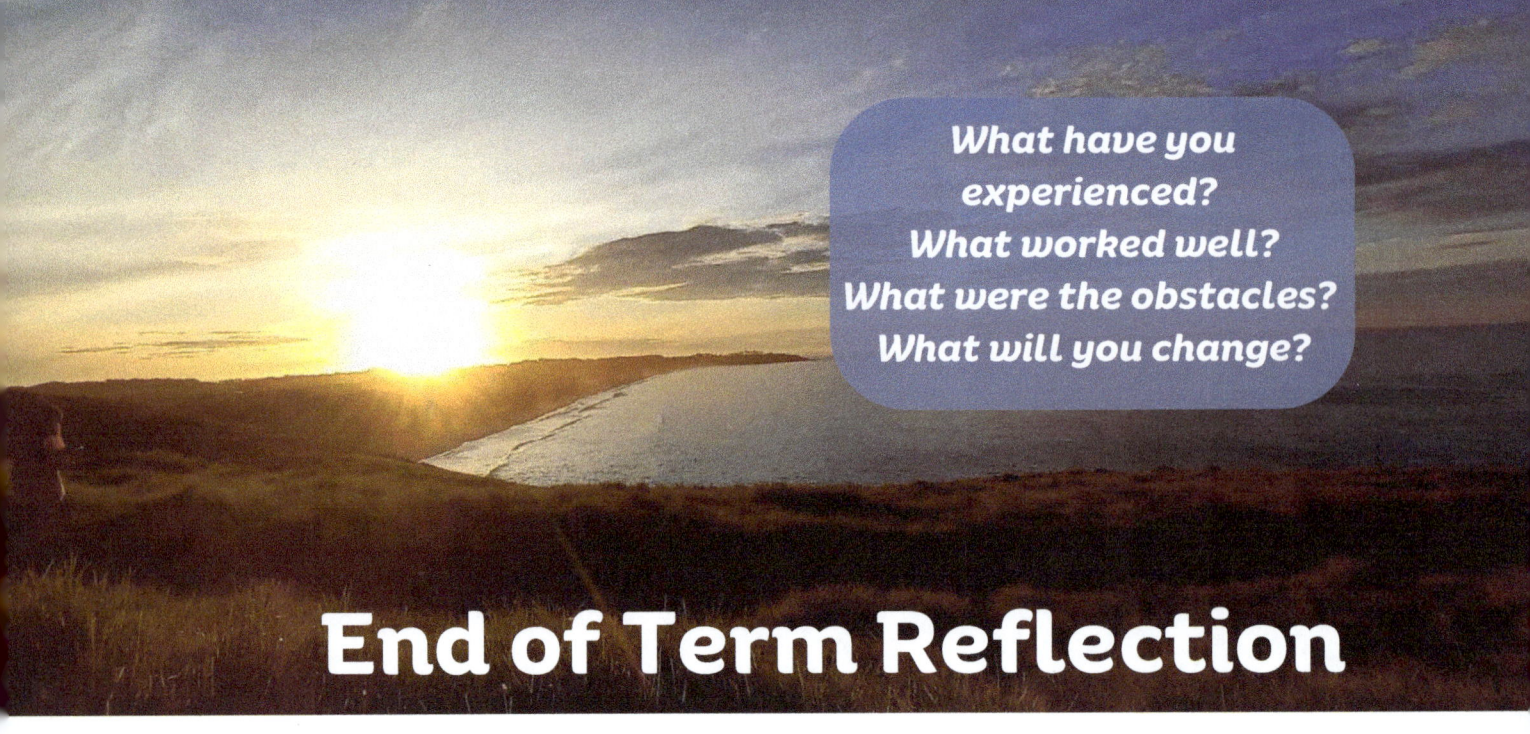

What have you experienced?
What worked well?
What were the obstacles?
What will you change?

End of Term Reflection

Think of this as your personal Warrant of Fitness—take time to regularly check in and ensure you're running smoothly.

- How would you rate your overall well-being this term? What factors contributed to your overall oranga
- What progress have you made towards your hauora goals?
- What areas do you need to focus on to improve your well-being?
- What specific goals or changes will you implement in the next term to enhance your oranga?

1. Me Kori Tonu - Be Active
   - How have you incorporated physical activity into your daily routine this term? What activities have you found most beneficial?
   - What worked well for you in staying active?
   - What challenges did you face in maintaining physical activity?
   - What changes or improvements will you make to your activity routine in the next term?

2. Me Whanaunga - Connect
   - How have you fostered or strengthened connections with hoamahi, ākonga and whānau this term?
   - What strategies helped you build and maintain these connections?
   - What obstacles did you encounter in staying connected?
   - What steps will you take to strengthen these connections in the future?

3. Me Aro Tonu - Taking Notice
   - How have you practiced mindfulness and stayed aware of your surroundings and feelings this term?
   - What mindfulness techniques or practices have you found most effective?
   - What difficulties have you experienced in staying mindful?
   - How will you enhance your mindfulness practices in the coming term?

4. Tukua - Giving
   - In what ways have you contributed to your community, school, or colleagues this term?
   - What acts of giving have been most rewarding for you?
   - Were there any barriers to giving that you encountered?
   - How can you increase your contributions and support in the next term?

5. Me Ako Tonu - Keep Learning
   - How have you engaged in learning new skills or knowledge this term? What have you learned about yourself?
   - What learning opportunities were most fulfilling or enjoyable?
   - Did you face any obstacles in pursuing learning goals?
   - What new learning goals will you set for yourself in the next term?

With daily, weekly, monthly, termly check ins, hopefully you will find yourself with new goals and find you enjoying the everyday and not waiting for the holidays to rest and reset.

A New Path, A New Purpose

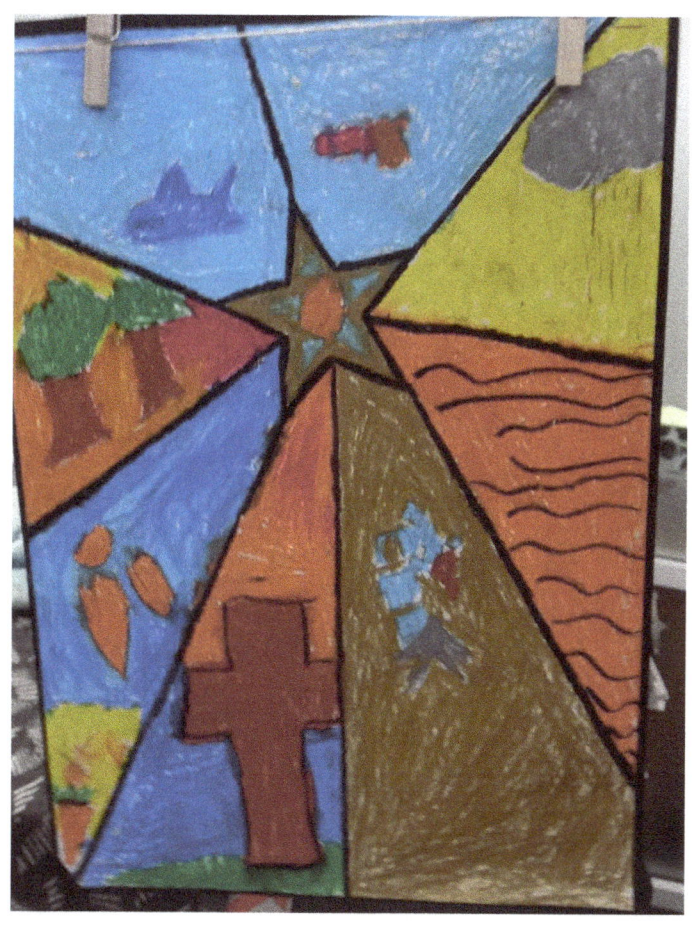

There was a time when she felt the weight
Of every lesson, every unanswered call,
Her heart pulling in too many directions,
Her mind cluttered with tasks and expectations,
The endless push to be more, give more,
Until there was nothing left for herself.
She stood on the edge of burnout,
A quiet exhaustion tugging at her core,
But she paused, let the noise settle,
Took a deep breath and chose a new path.
It wasn't easy to step away,
From the faces that once defined her,
From the rhythm she had known so long.
But in the space of uncertainty,
She found herself again—
Stronger, clearer, with a purpose that now feels like home.
Her days are different now.
There's time to breathe, to reflect,
To be present in the moments that matter.
She works with joy and intention,
A career shaped by balance,
Not driven by the rush of more.
She's found her confidence
In the quiet spaces between tasks,
In the pause before saying yes.
Her life, a harmony of work and rest,
Of giving and receiving,
She is whole again,
And this time, she knows—
She will never lose herself in the hurry.

Erin Steel 2021

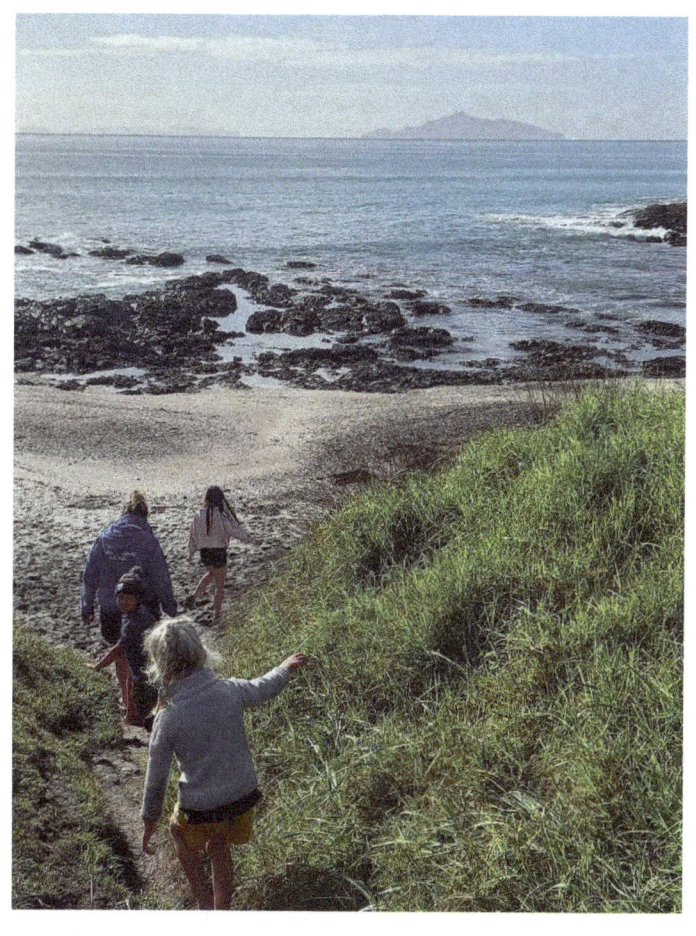

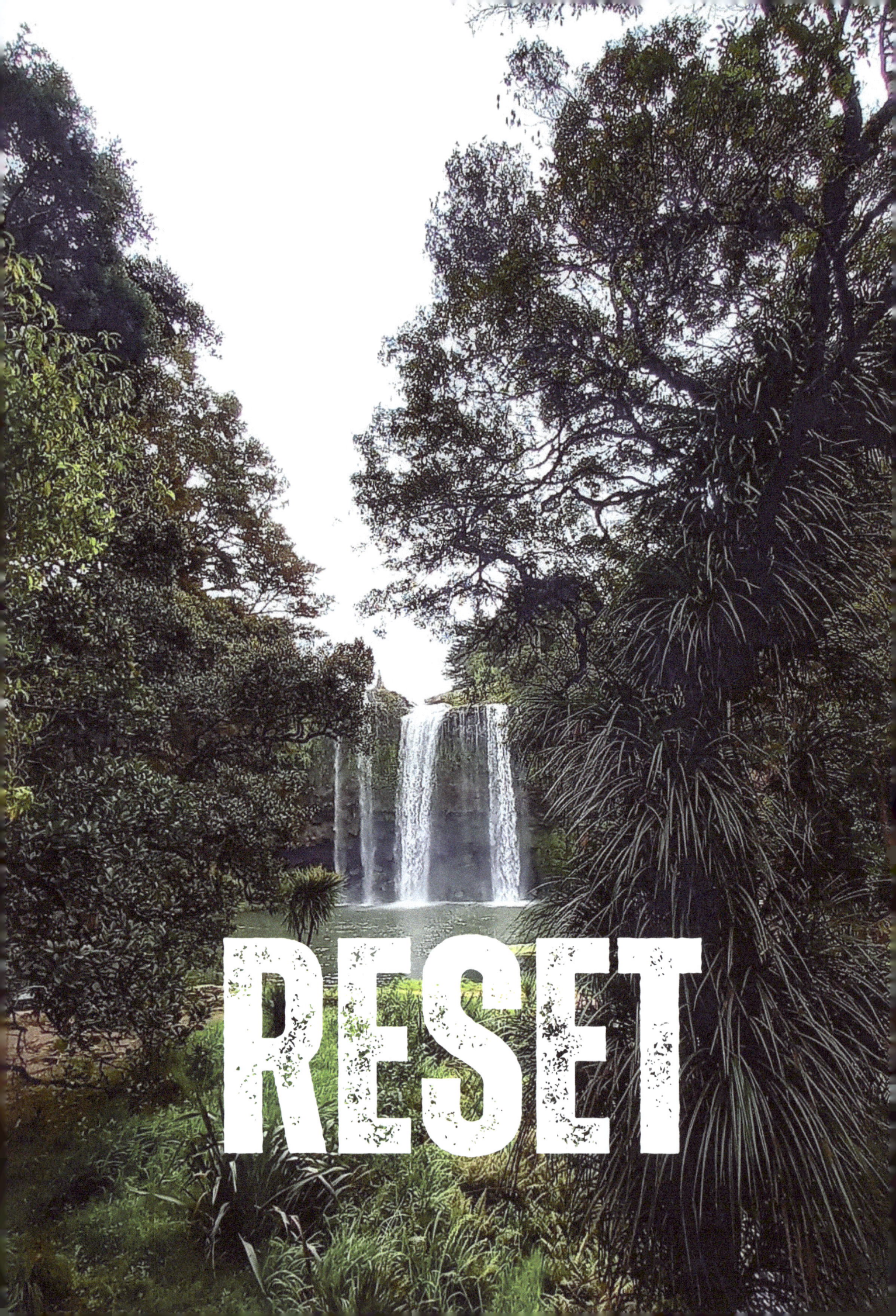

Mindfulness Month Reflection

I loved my newly found and nurtured habit,
A daily practice of mindfulness,
A gift I had given to myself—
A pause, a breath,
A chance to tune in to the stillness that lay beneath.

As Mindfulness Month came to a close,
I sat in quiet reflection,
Grateful for the shared journey we had walked together.
Each moment, each gesture of support,
Tautoko that lifted us as we explored new depths
Of self-awareness and community.

To the organisers, their vision had ignited this path,
Their tireless dedication shaped each day.
They wove workshops, conversations,
And the kind of learning that took root deep,
Inspiring us all to carry the light of mindfulness forward.

To every supporter—
Your kindness had been our foundation,
Allowing us to reach further,
To spark hope, to uplift others.
Through your generosity,
The seeds of mindfulness were planted in fertile ground.
Together, we had touched the quiet power of presence,
Found strength in small moments of calm,
And wove new connections—
Within ourselves, with our whānau, with each other.
As we closed this chapter,
We carried this awareness into the future.

Mindfulness didn't end there—
It became a daily practice,
A gift we continued to give to ourselves and to those around us.
And next year, when the month returns,
Join us again.
Let's deepen this journey,
Spread its message wider,
And continue to nurture the hauora of our community,
One mindful breath at a time.

Erin Steel 2023

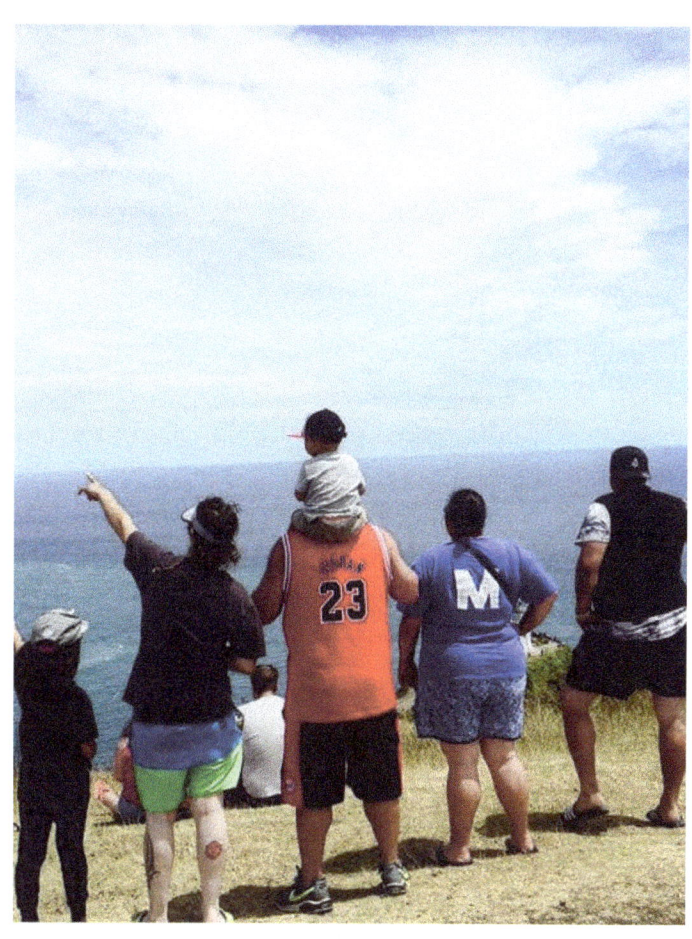

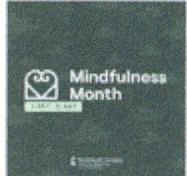

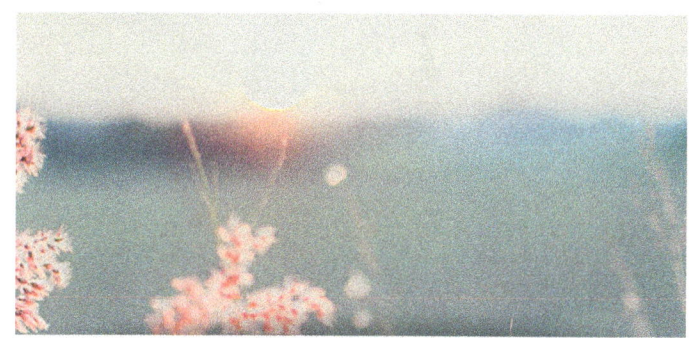

He aroha whakatō, he aroha puta mai
If kindness is sown, then kindness is received.

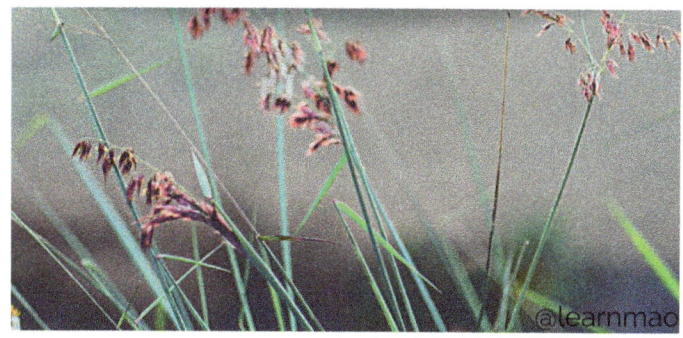

SMART GOALS – Here's how to get started:

1. *Specific*
Begin by identifying a clear and specific goal. Instead of a vague intention like "I want to exercise more," opt for something like, "I will go for a 30-minute hikoī (walk) three times a week." Specific goals provide clarity and direction, making it easier to take action.

2. *Measurable*
Measurable goals allow you to track your progress. This could mean setting a goal to read one book per month on a topic you're passionate about or aiming to complete a certain number of professional development hours within the school year. By quantifying your goals, you can celebrate your achievements along the way, which reinforces your commitment.

3. *Achievable*
While it's important to challenge yourself, ensure your goals are realistic. If you're new to walking, don't set a goal to complete a half marathon in a month. Instead, aim for a 5km or a 10km within a few weeks and gradually increase your distance. Achievable goals build confidence and keep you motivated.

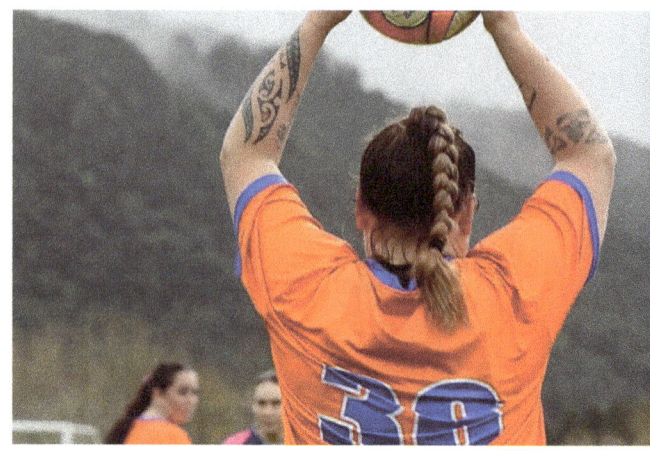

4. *Relevant*
Choose goals that resonate with your personal interests and professional aspirations. If you have a passion for art, consider setting a goal to incorporate more creative projects into your teaching. This not only enriches your own life but also inspires your ākonga (students) and enhances their learning experiences.

5. *Time-bound*
Set a deadline for your goals to create a sense of urgency. For instance, "I will complete a weekend workshop on mindfulness practices by the end of the term." Having a timeline keeps you focused and accountable.

Putting It All Together
Let's say you're passionate about your māra kai (garden) and want to integrate this into your classroom. A SMART goal could be:
Specific: I will create a small garden project with my ākonga.
Measurable: We will plant five different types of seeds and track their growth.
Achievable: I will dedicate one class per week to garden activities.
Relevant: This project will enhance my ākonga and their understanding of science and responsibility.
Time-bound: We will complete the project by the end of the term.

Call to action - share your SMART goals with your hoamahi and create a supportive community that encourages personal growth.

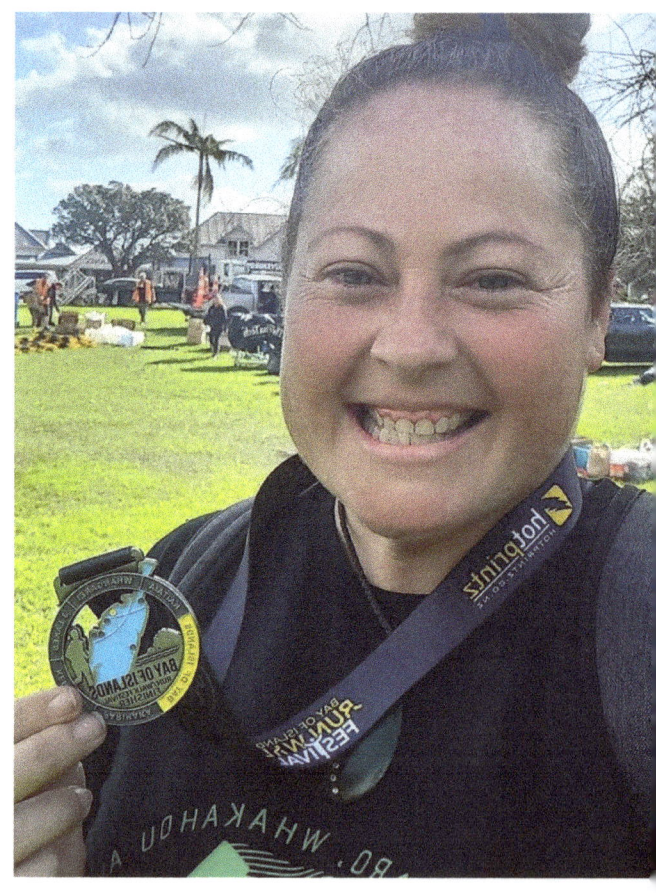

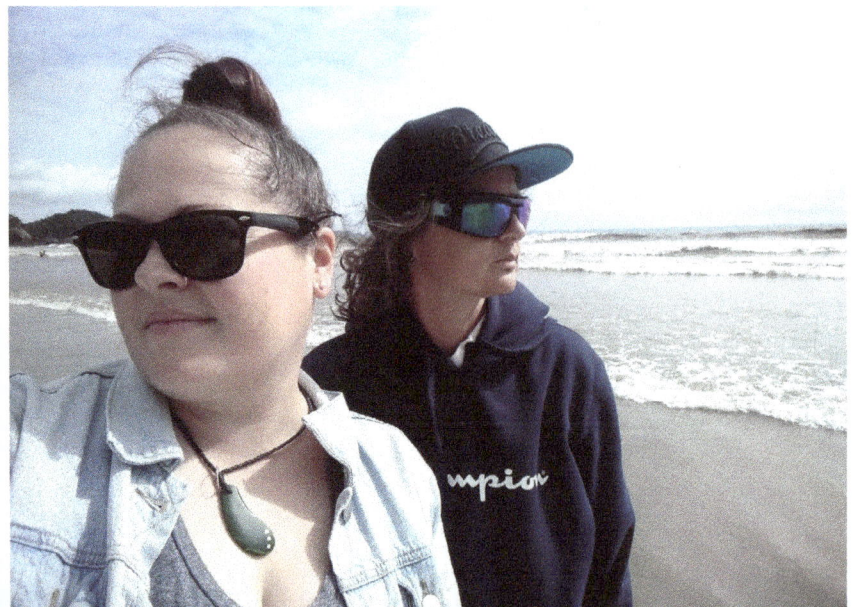

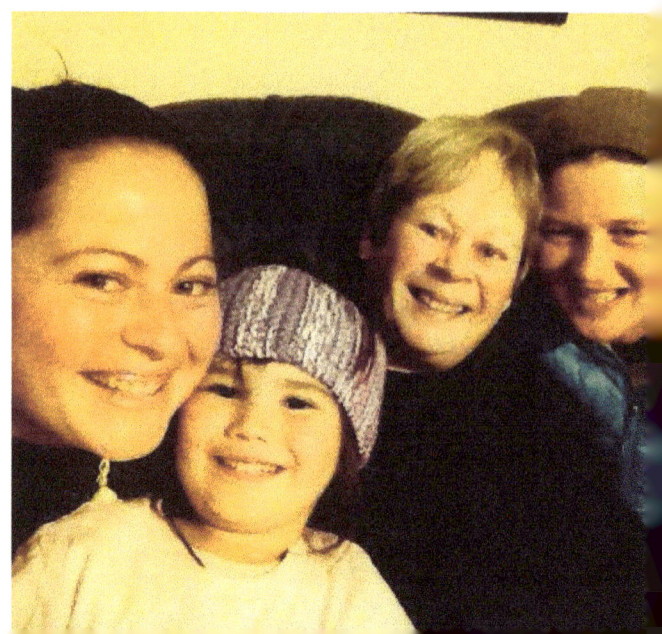

Want to make small sustainable changes? Develop Effective Habits

INSPIRED BY KAREN TUI BOYES

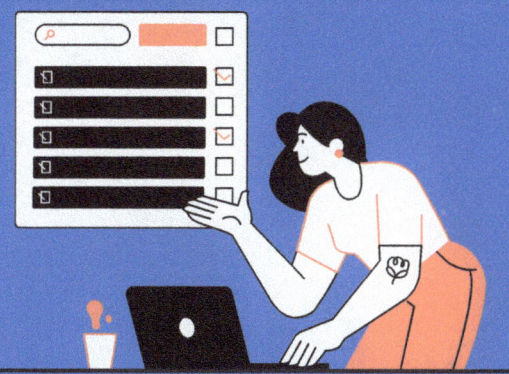

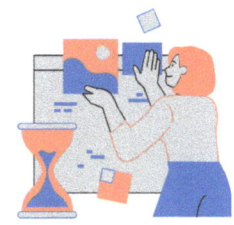

Start Small and Be Consistent

Consistency is key, commit to practicing the habit daily to reinforce its development.

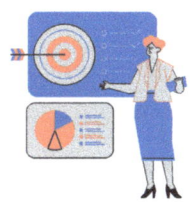

Set Clear and Specific Goals

Make your goals measurable, achievable and relevant to keep yourself motivated.

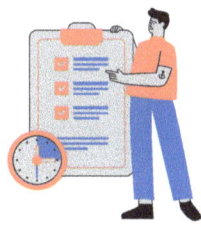

Track Your Progress

Keep a habit tracker or journal to monitor your daily or weekly commitment to the habit.

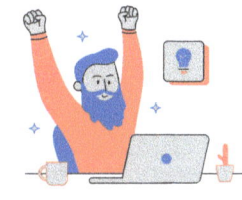

Use Positive Reinforcement

Celebrate small wins and reward yourself for sticking to the habit. Positive reinforcement encourages continued behaviour.

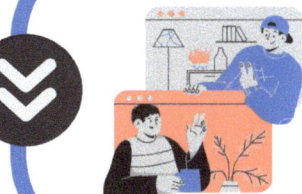

Build a Support System

Share your habit-building journey with friends or family who can encourage and support you.

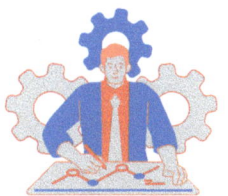

Focus on the WHY

Understand the reasons behind developing the habit and its positive impact on your life.

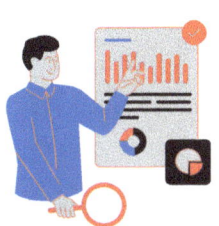

Learn from Setbacks

Accept that setbacks are a part of the habit-building process. Analyse the reasons for setbacks and use them as opportunities to improve.

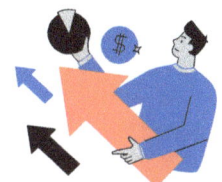

Review and Adjust

Visualise yourself performing the habit effortlessly and achieving your goals.

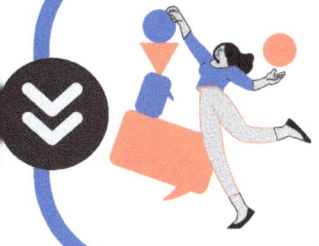

Implement Habit Stacking

Attach the new habit to an existing one that is already well-established. This way, you build on an existing routine to develop new habits seamlessly.

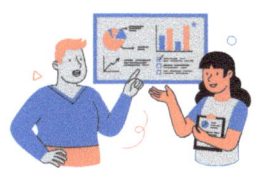

Visualise Success

Regularly review your habit-building journey and assess the effectiveness of the habit.

39

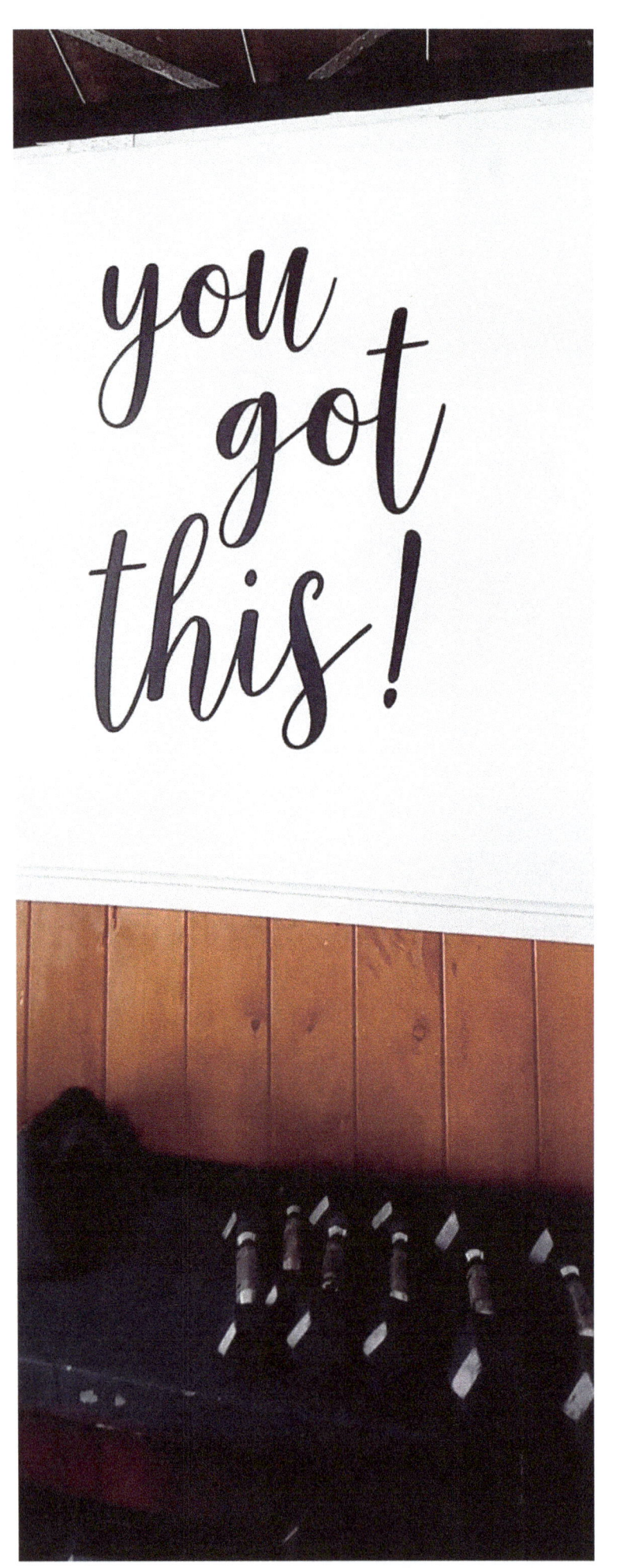

Take a moment today to pause and reflect. Think about the journey you've been on—how far you've come and the lives you've touched. Sometimes the path feels extremely challenging. Know you've got the strength, resilience and perseverance to keep going.

Find your momentum, even the smallest steps lead to big progress. Celebrate those little wins—whether it's a breakthrough with a student, a new strategy that worked, or simply showing up as your best self.

Unlock your confidence, remember, no one does it quite like you! Your unique gifts, your passion and your commitment to your tamariki and ākonga make a difference every day.

Trust yourself and your instincts. Keep moving forward when self-doubt creeps in, take a breath, reflect and remind yourself that you're on the right path. With each challenge, you grow stronger, more capable and more impactful.

Believe in yourself - because we do! You are valued. You are inspiring. You are making a difference. Ka mau te wehi!

#YouGotThis #Confidence #MomentumMatters
#ReflectAndGrow #HeKākanoAhau

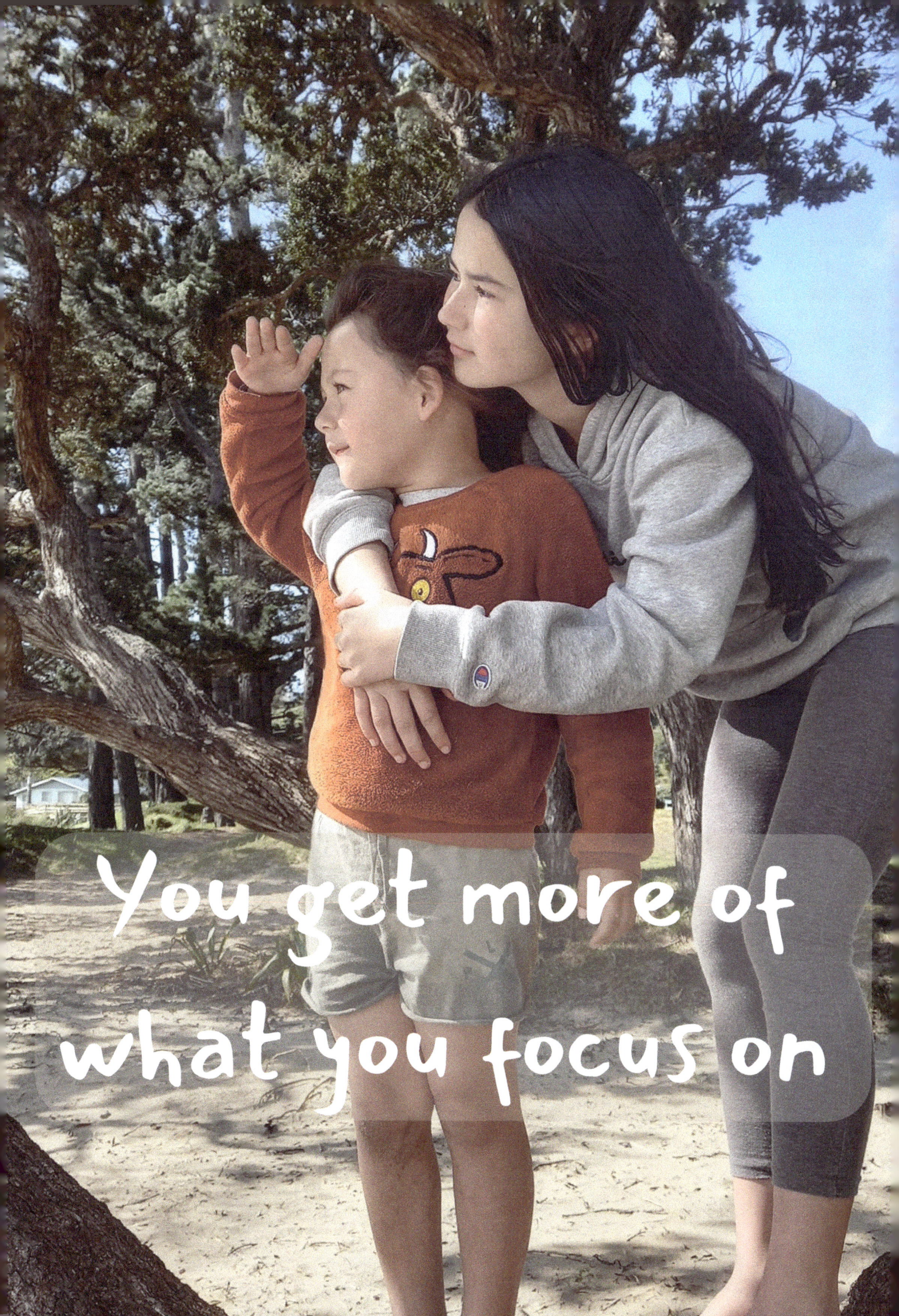

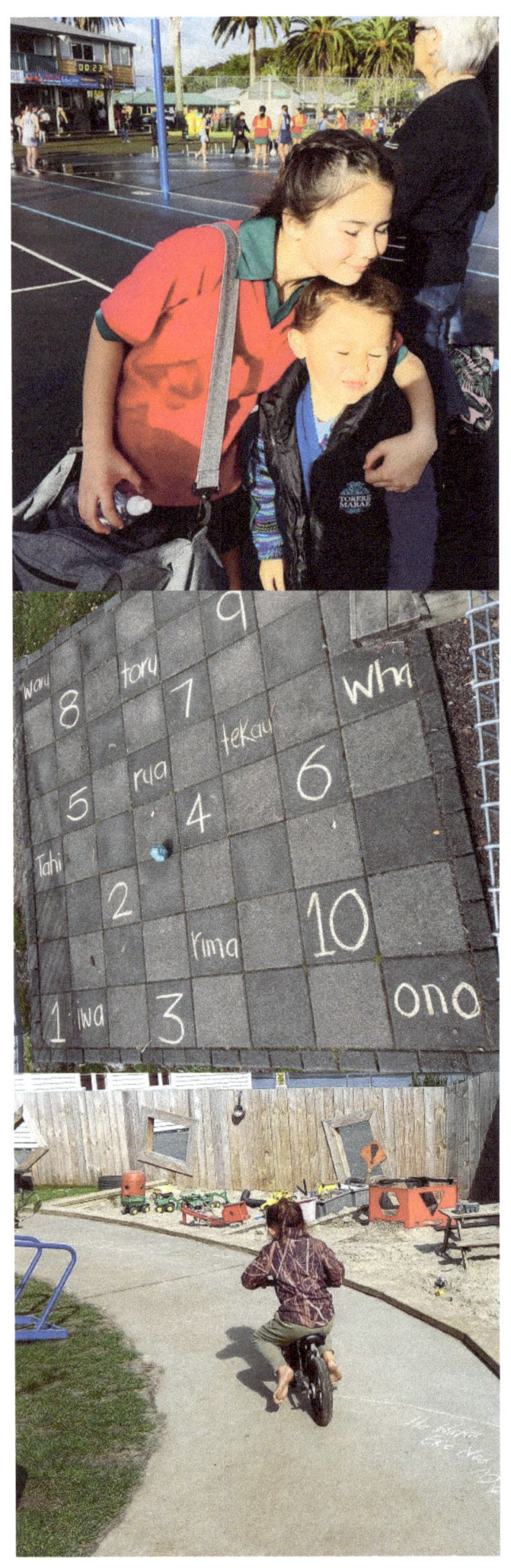

Revamp Your Health and Physical Education Curriculum:
Infusing Oranga into Lifelong Learning. Let's inspire our students to embrace lifelong learning through a focus on Oranga—well-being of the whole self!

Health and Physical Education (HPE) is more than just keeping students active; it's about nurturing their oranga—their physical, mental, social and emotional well-being. A strong HPE plan fosters confidence, encourages critical thinking, and embeds a lifelong love for movement and wellness. But what does such a plan look like in practice?

At the heart of an effective HPE plan is the goal of building students' confidence and hauora (well-being), empowering them with the skills, knowledge, and enthusiasm to engage in movement as part of their everyday lives. Whether through outdoor experiences, play-based activities, kapa haka, or traditional sports, the plan should connect to Te Whare Tapa Whā—the four dimensions of well-being—so students see movement as an integral part of their oranga.

A robust HPE plan encourages students to reflect on their own health and think critically about the world around them. Discussions and activities rooted in whakawhanaungatanga can help students understand the importance of physical activity, not only for their own well-being but for the well-being of their whānau and communities. This can be achieved through learning opportunities that tie in with local customs, cultural activities like Matariki celebrations, and societal challenges.

By using the underlying concepts of the HPE curriculum, educators can guide students to make meaningful connections between their health and their environment. Lessons should link to students' lived experiences, showing them how the skills and knowledge they gain in HPE can lead to positive changes in their own lives and those around them. Connecting to whenua through outdoor education, or diving for kai moana, adds layers of cultural relevance and strengthens their oranga by grounding them in their heritage.

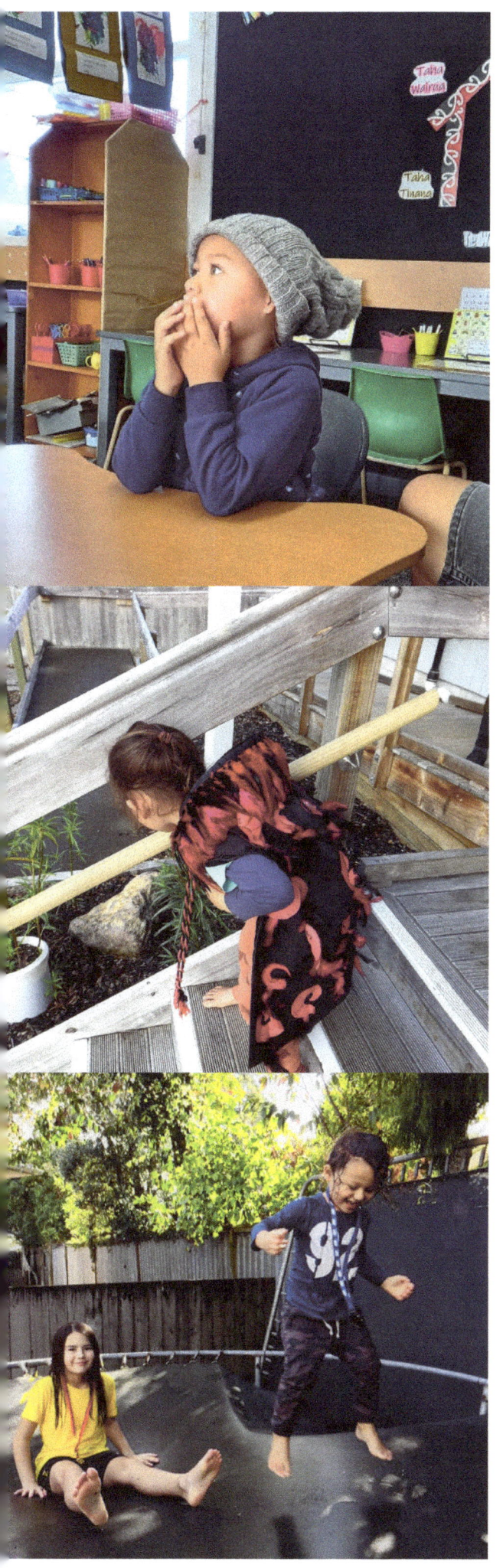

An effective HPE plan places ākonga at its center. Allowing students to co-construct their learning experiences—whether designing activities or reflecting on their progress—encourages them to take ownership of their oranga. Regular reflections enable ākonga to articulate their successes, challenges and personal growth, making them more invested in their lifelong well-being journey.

For any HPE plan to truly succeed, educators must be fully engaged. This means co-creating lessons with ākonga and being passionate about the impact that a holistic approach to health and physical education can have on their oranga. Kaiako should feel empowered to adapt activities to meet the needs of their ākonga, fostering a whānau atmosphere where everyone feels valued and included.

Collaboration with the wider community is key. Whether inviting local kaumātua to share knowledge, partnering with marae for noho experiences, or working with local sports clubs, involving community experts enriches the HPE experience and deepens ākonga connection to their cultural and social environments.

Incorporating cross-curricular links is also vital. Combining HPE with subjects like Te Reo Māori or whakapapa fosters an integrated approach to learning, helping ākonga see the connections between movement, history and identity.

Ākonga leadership should be encouraged as part of the plan. Whether setting personal health goals, leading class challenges, or organising community events, ākonga gain confidence when given the chance to manaaki themselves and others. Allowing ākonga to take lead of their own oranga helps them develop lifelong healthy habits and a sense of responsibility toward their well-being.

Embrace innovation in your HPE planning—your ākonga, their whānau and your community will thank you for it!

> Creativity, collaboration and a focus on oranga, educators can build a curriculum that not only meets educational needs, it inspires lifelong healthy habits for ākonga.
> When we connect the HPE curriculum to real-life experiences, we empower ākonga voice and we create an environment where oranga thrives.

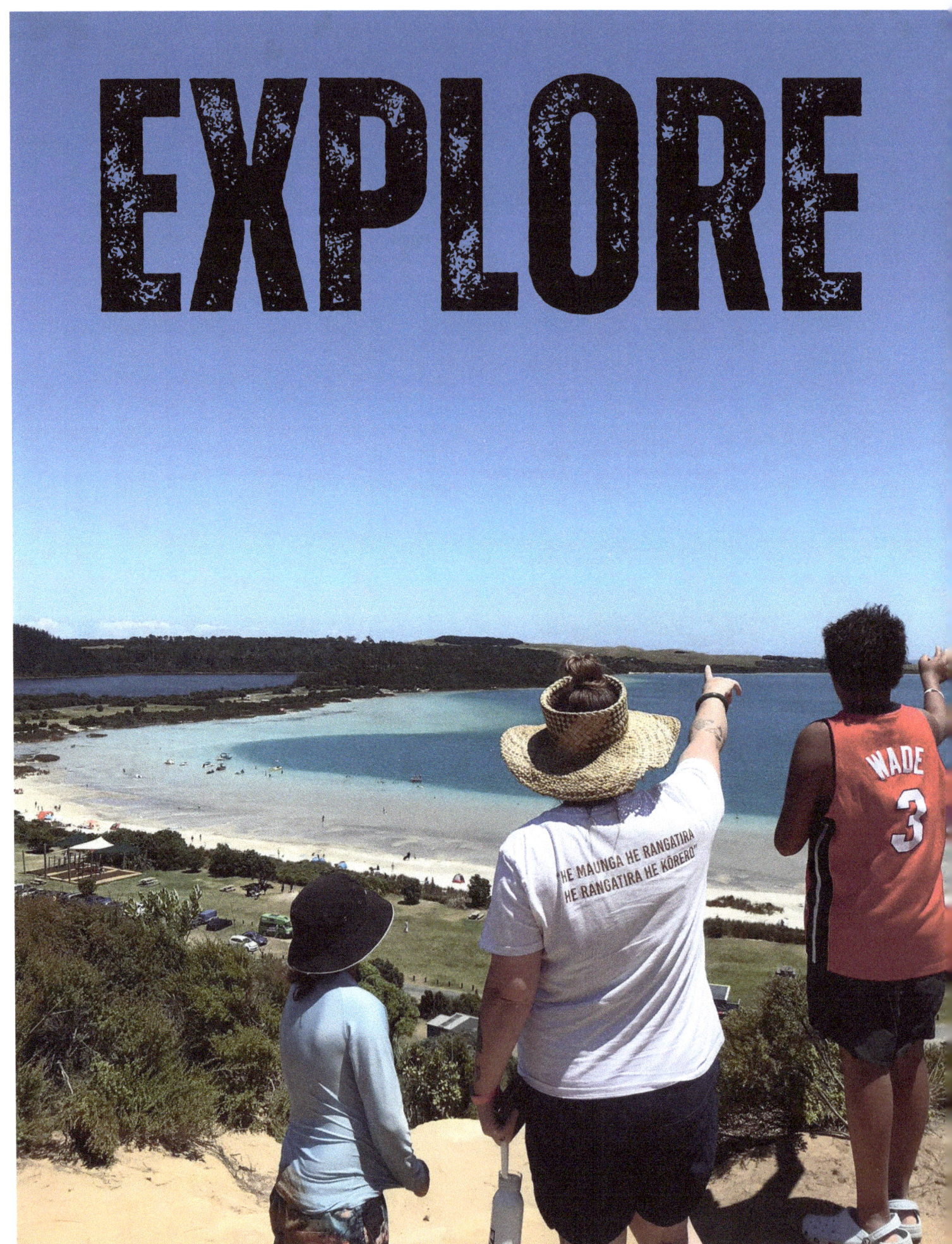

"He aha te kai o te rangatira? He kōrero, he kōrero, he kōrero."
"What is the food of the leader? It is knowledge, it is communication, it is dialogue."

TALKING STEMS

This whakataukī emphasises the importance of dialogue and communication in leadership and learning. It encourages reflective and engaging discussions as a means of nourishing the mind and fostering growth and understanding.

As educators, we know that Health and Physical Education extends beyond mere physical activity; it delves into critical domains like mental health, nutrition and personal well-being. However, facilitating and sustaining meaningful dialogue in these areas often poses challenges for educators.

You can carefully craft talking stems to encourage specific types of responses, such as elaboration, clarification, agreement, or disagreement. Providing a framework for communication, talking stems empower students to express their thoughts more effectively.

Talking stems ensure that all students have a voice in the discussion, regardless of their confidence level or communication skills, create a supportive environment where every student feels valued and heard.

HPE encompasses extremely important and often sensitive topics related to mental health, nutrition and personal well-being. Intentional talking stems help students articulate their thoughts on complex subjects.

Prompting students to explain their reasoning or provide evidence for their opinions, talking stems encourage deeper reflection and critical analysis. Enhancing students' ability to think critically about health-related issues and make informed decisions in their own lives.

Talking stems promote respectful reflective dialogue and active listening, creating a supportive learning environment where students feel comfortable expressing their ideas and engaging with their peers.

Incorporating talking stems teachers not only facilitate meaningful discussions but also gather critical information to inform and enhance their instructional planning. This continuous feedback loop ensures that teaching strategies are responsive to student needs.

Introduce talking stems gradually, modeling how to use them effectively and providing opportunities for students to practice using them in pairs or small groups before implementing them in whole-class discussions.

Using your mode of communication, share and display a list of common talking stems to serve as a reference for students during discussions or turn it into a bookmark for individual reference.

Encourage students to reflect on their use of talking stems and provide feedback on their peers' contributions. This promotes metacognitive awareness and helps students refine their communication skills over time.

Creating Impact by Facilitating Meaningful Dialogue

TALKING STEMS

- To improve my mental well-being, I plan to...
- I believe personal well-being includes... because...
- To raise awareness about [health issue], I suggest we...
- I agree with [student's name]'s point about [activity] because...
- I respectfully disagree with [student's name] because I believe...
- I feel that [type of physical activity] is important because...
- To support my friends' mental well-being, I could...
- In my experience, [physical activity] helps me feel... because...

When we integrate talking stems into HPE lessons we are enhancing student dialogue, fostering inclusivity, developing communication skills, encouraging critical thinking and building a positive classroom culture. By providing a communication framework, talking stems deepen student engagement with content and each other, ultimately improving learning outcomes and creating a more enriching educational experience.

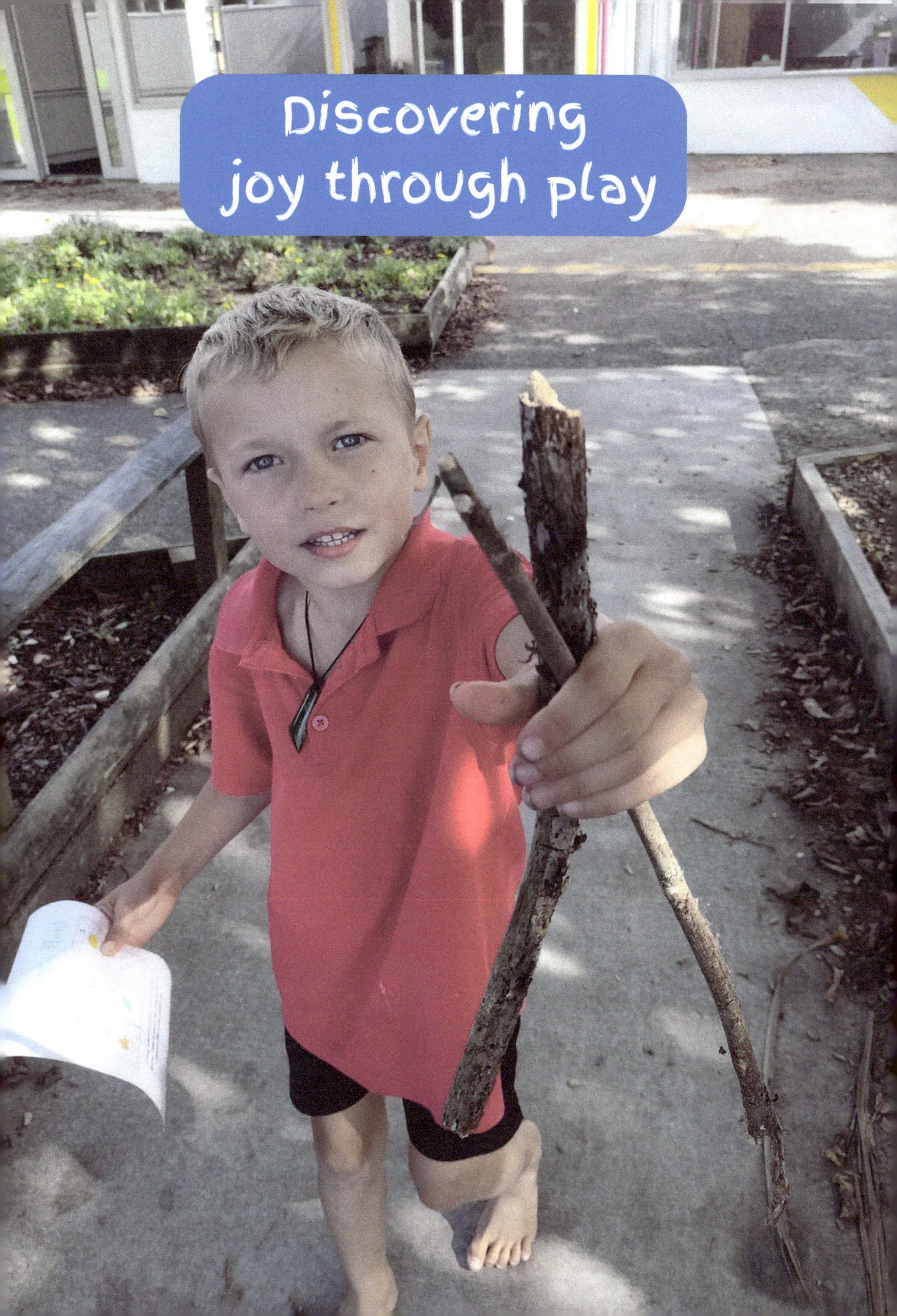

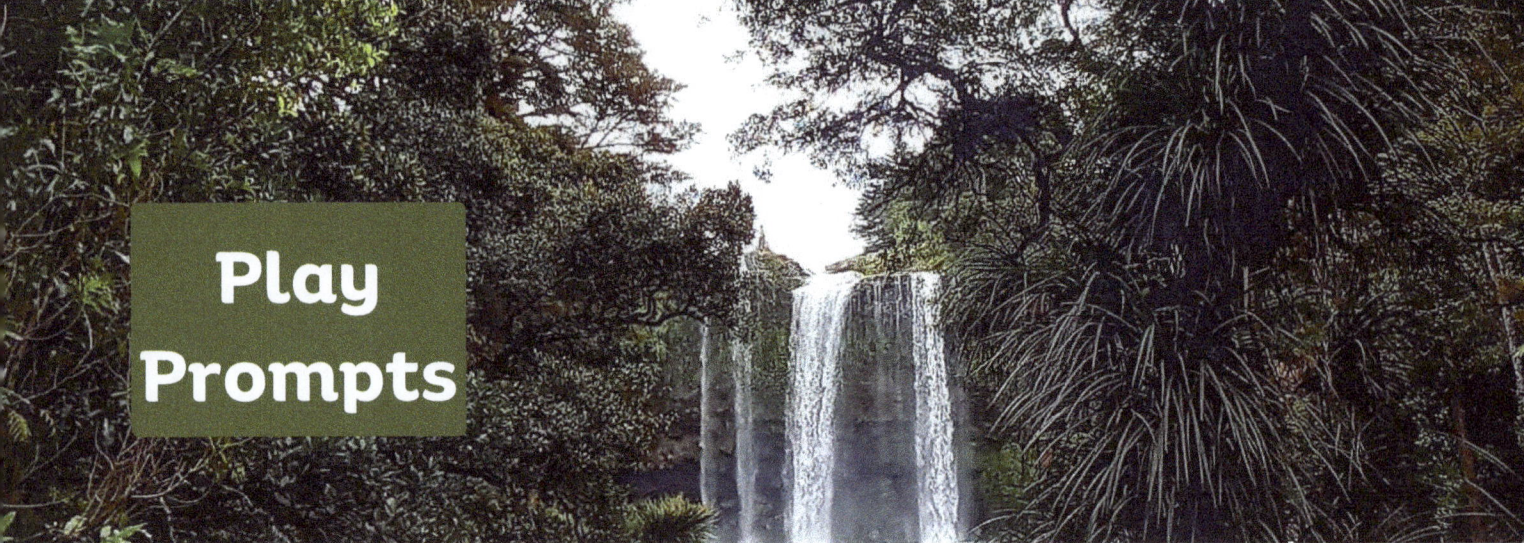

Play Prompts

As adults, play often looks different from childhood games, it can still be a vital part of well-being and mental health. For kaiako, who give so much to their students, play can be a way to reconnect with joy, creativity and movement.

1 RECONNECT WITH CHILDHOOD PLAY

Think back to a game or activity you loved as a child. How did it make you feel? Find a way to bring that activity into your life this week, even if it's modified for adulthood. It could be skipping, hopscotch, or building something with your hands.
Reflect: How does revisiting this childhood joy change your mood and energy?

2 MOVE PLAYFULLY

Choose a type of movement that feels playful to you, whether it's dancing in your living room, kicking a ball around, or trying a new workout that feels fun instead of structured. Make it about enjoyment, not performance.
Reflect: How does moving your body in a playful way impact your stress levels or mindset?

3 CREATIVE PLAYSMISSION

Pick a creative activity that you don't often make time for, like drawing, painting, or playing a musical instrument. Don't worry about the outcome—just focus on the process of creation.
Reflect: What emotions come up when you create something just for fun? How does this feel different from your usual routine?

4 SOCIAL PLAY

Organise a playful activity with colleagues—something light and fun like a team-building game, a short quiz, or a collaborative art project. Even playing board games or charades during a break can spark laughter and connection.
Reflect: How does shared play with others influence your relationships and sense of community at work?

5 OUTDOOR EXPLORATION

Spend some time outdoors, exploring nature in a playful way. Try going on a spontaneous adventure: climb a tree, splash in a puddle, or go barefoot on the grass. Let go of adult inhibitions and enjoy the simplicity of the moment.
Reflect: How does being playful in nature affect your mood and mental clarity?

6 CHALLENGE YOURSELF WITH FUN

-Try something new that you've never done before, but have always been curious about—whether it's a new hobby, sport, or game. Approach it with a playful attitude, focusing on fun rather than success.
Reflect: What does trying something new teach you about yourself? How does it feel to be a beginner at play?

7 INCORPORATE PLAY INTO YOUR DAY

Turn an everyday task, like walking or tidying up, into a playful challenge. For example, count how many steps it takes to get from one end of your classroom to the other, or see how many items you can pick up in a minute.
Reflect: How can adding an element of play to routine tasks make them more enjoyable and less stressful?

"Giving yourself permission to play, you can reignite a sense of joy and connection to the present moment. What brings you joy may look different now than it did as a child, but the impact of play—on creativity, mental health and emotional well-being—is just as powerful. Take time to explore what play looks like for you today and share that joy with those around you."

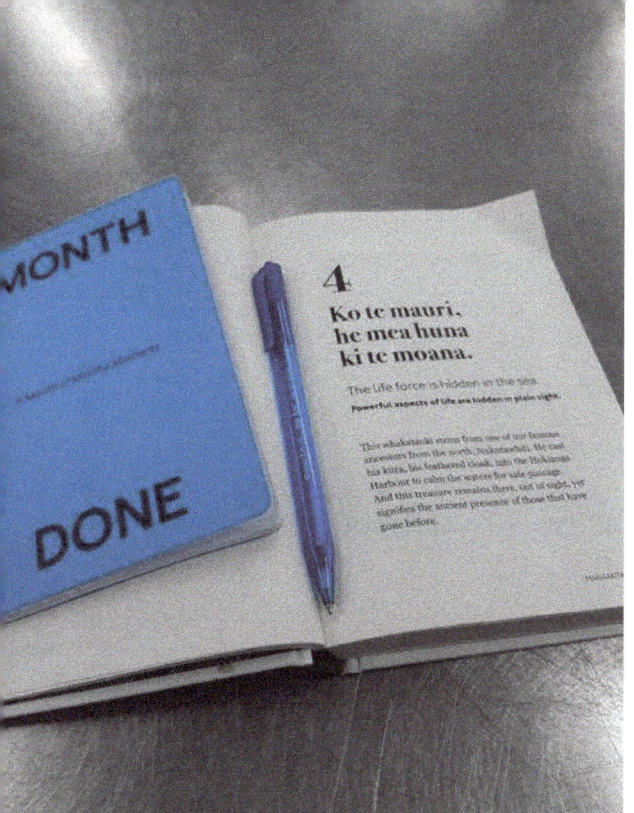
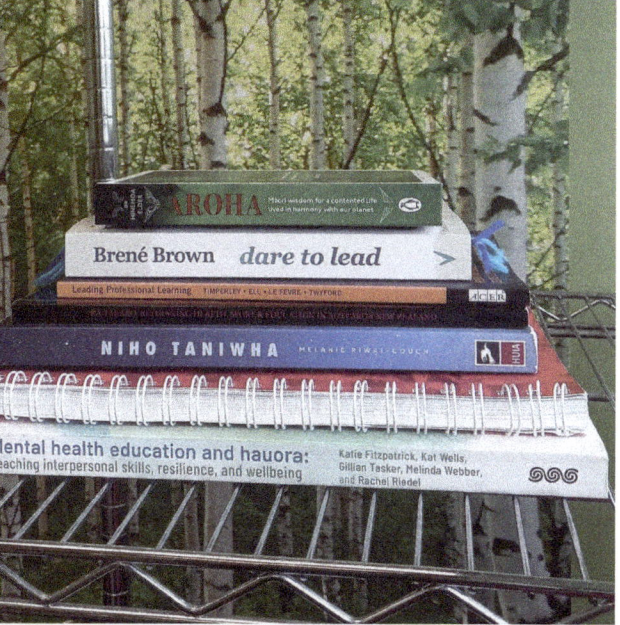
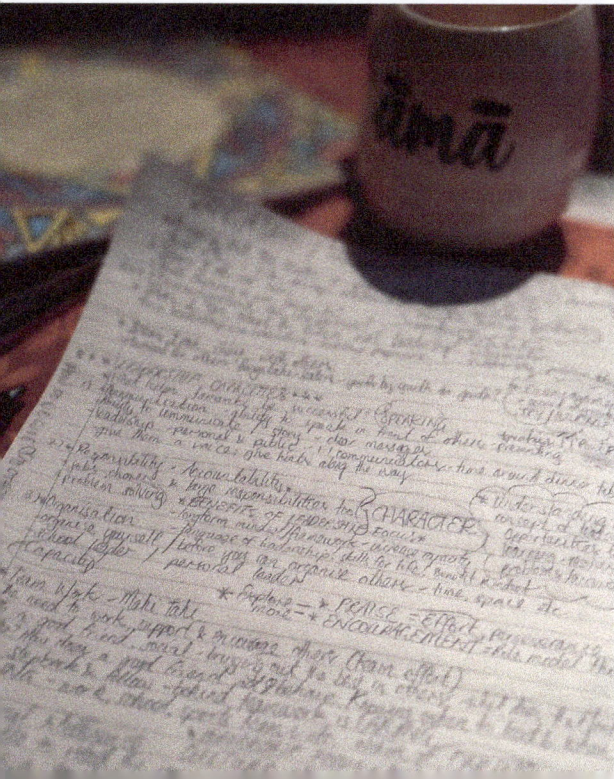

STRENGTHENING CONFIDENCE

Emotional Intelligence

Strengthening Confidence

Supporting kaiako to regulate their emotions. Why it matters in education.

Being a kaiako is both a privilege and a challenge. Each day, kaiako engage with ākonga, colleagues and whānau while managing various responsibilities. At the heart of this mahi lies a crucial skill: emotional regulation. The ability to understand, manage and respond to emotions in a healthy way is key to thriving in the classroom. Emotional regulation not only impacts kaiako well-being but also significantly influences student learning and the overall atmosphere of the school.

Creating a positive learning environment

Kaiako set the tone for the classroom. When they can manage their emotions effectively, they create a safe, supportive and calm environment where ākonga feel comfortable and ready to learn. Classrooms are dynamic places where emotions can shift quickly, whether due to a challenging lesson, a student's behavior, or external pressures. By regulating emotions, kaiako can respond to these shifts with patience and empathy, ensuring that their reactions do not escalate tensions but instead foster a sense of calm.

Kaiako who can remain composed under stress, model emotional stability for ākonga, teaching them how to embrace and sit with their own emotions. This encourages a positive classroom culture where respect and understanding become the norm.

Enhancing teacher well-being

Teaching is demanding, both mentally and emotionally. Without the ability to regulate emotions, kaiako may find themselves overwhelmed by stress, frustration, or burnout. Emotional regulation serves as a form of self-care, helping kaiako manage their own well-being while balancing the needs of others.

When teachers take time to pause, reflect and respond to their emotions with awareness, they are better equipped to prevent burnout and maintain their passion for teaching. Strategies like deep breathing, mindfulness and taking regular breaks to recharge can make a significant difference in how kaiako feel at the end of the day. Self-regulation enables kaiako to show up as their best selves, not only for their students but also for themselves and their whānau.

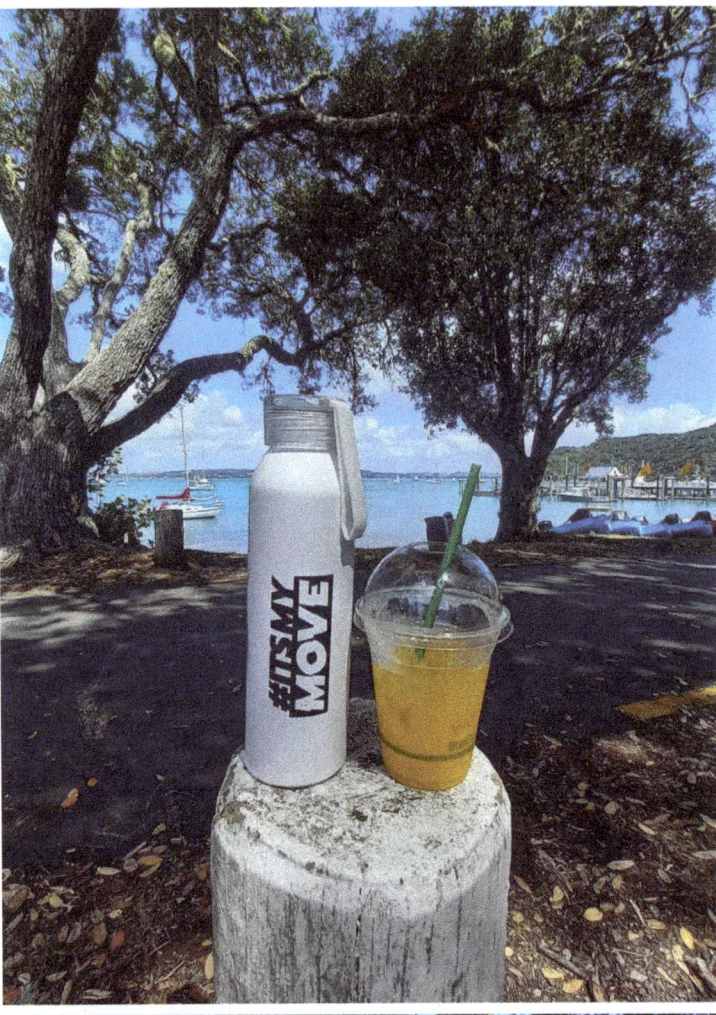

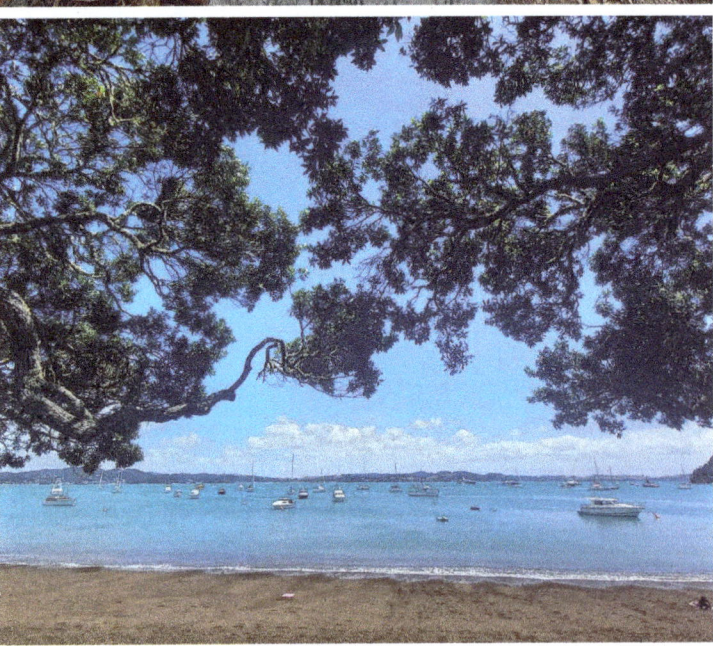

Building stronger relationships with whānau

Emotional regulation also plays a key role in how kaiako engage with whānau. Positive communication with parents and caregivers is fundamental to student success and kaiako who can manage their emotions are better equipped to navigate challenging conversations.

When kaiako regulate their emotions, they can approach whānau discussions with empathy and understanding, even in difficult situations. This creates opportunities for constructive conversations focused on finding solutions for ākonga rather than becoming defensive or reactive. Strong relationships with whānau are built on mutual trust and respect, which emotional regulation helps to nurture.

Practical strategies for kaiako to regulate their emotions

- Mindful pauses or taking a few moments throughout the day to breathe and center yourself can help reset your emotional state. When emotions begin to rise, pausing to take deep breaths or practicing mindfulness can make a world of difference.
- Reflective practice at the end of each day. Take time to reflect on emotional triggers and how you responded. This helps increase self-awareness and provides insight into how you can improve your emotional regulation.
- Boundaries and breaks prioritise setting boundaries between work and personal life.
- Make time for breaks during the day, even if they are short. A brief walk or time outdoors can do wonders for emotional balance.

Emotional Literacy

- Take time to recognise and name your emotions. Being able to identify what you're feeling can help you address those emotions in healthy ways, rather than letting them build up.
- Self-compassion, be kind to yourself. Teaching is challenging and it's important to give yourself grace when things don't go perfectly. Self-compassion strengthens emotional resilience.
- Peer support, don't hesitate to reach out to trusted colleagues when you need support. Talking through emotions with others can help release tension and provide valuable perspective.

For kaiako, regulating emotions is not just an individual skill but a powerful tool that can change classrooms, improve student outcomes and facilitates a culture of well-being. By understanding and managing emotions, teachers create environments where ākonga can thrive, relationships can flourish and the challenges of teaching can be met with resilience and grace. Embracing emotional regulation is key to not only sustaining a long and rewarding career, ensuring that kaiako can continue to make a positive impact on the lives of their students and communities.

Whakawhetai Gratitude - a daily practice

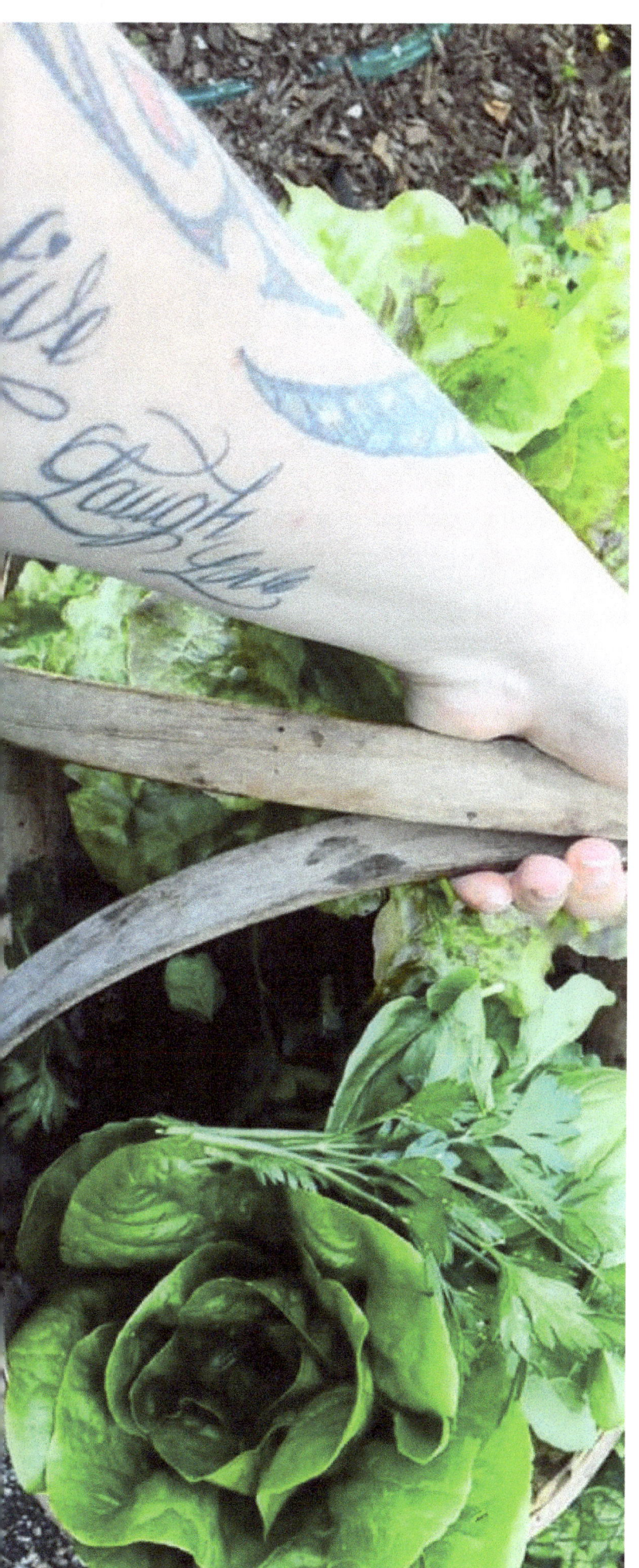

Each day begins with a breath—
a quiet invitation to be here, now,
to open my eyes and really see.
The stillness of dawn, the soft rustle of leaves in the wind outside my window, remind me to pause, to embrace the world around me.

In the noticing,
my hauora finds its balance.
Te Taha Tinana—my body—
feels the rhythm of my steps,
grounded in the earth beneath.
Te Taha Wairua—my spirit—
lifts in moments of awe,
anchored in something larger
than this day alone.

I practice awareness,
honoring Te Taha Hinengaro—my mind
— as it slows, letting go of the rush, the need to be elsewhere.

And in this stillness,
Te Taha Whānau—my connections—
grow deeper, as I learn to listen,
to truly be present with those I love.

Gratitude in every corner,
in every small act,
shapes this practice.
A daily unfolding
of well-being,
from moments of awareness—
a life lived noticing,
embracing,
becoming whole.

Erin Steel 2022

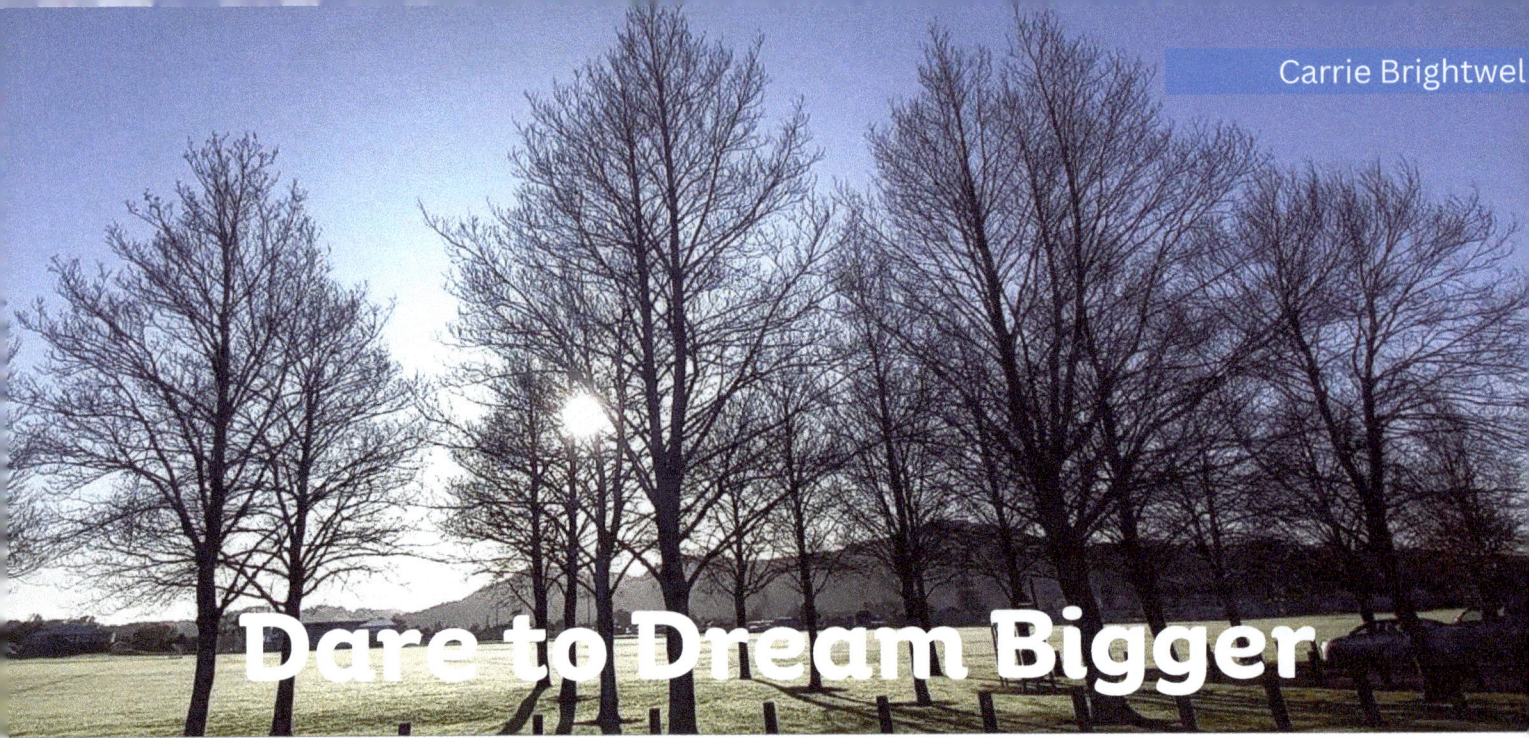

Dare to Dream Bigger

Carrie Brightwel

From my observations and experience, many of those who are living day-to-day with disrupting feelings such as frustration, lack of fulfilment, boredom, misery, or anger, with a sense of wanting more, do so because they are settling for a version of life that is not aligned to their true desires, purpose or full potential. Instead, they are settling for what they have been told they should have or think they've been given.

I'm guessing that you're here because:
- You want to change and have something different for yourself and your family.
- You want a more positive, invigorating and fulfilling experience of life.
- You want to reconnect to who you really are and to that essence that is bigger than you.
- Be purposeful, live out your full potential and contribute to the world and humanity

Many traditional forms of therapy or self-help will look at taking you from a negative state to a neutral one.

If you focus on neutrality and mediocracy all you will ever be is neutral and mediocre.

You can choose mediocrity or you can choose greatness, fulfillment, purpose and success. I will share with you today the formula that I teach, guide and support so that you can start to live a life you bloody love.

Hope, excitement, motivation, confidence, drive, enthusiasm, joy, love, desire, peace, contentment, liberation, freedom, fulfilment - these are some examples of what is possible.

I want you to become the greatest version of yourself. One that you don't even know is possible. So, rather than bringing you from negative to neutral, let's shift you from wherever you are now to great and then even greater.

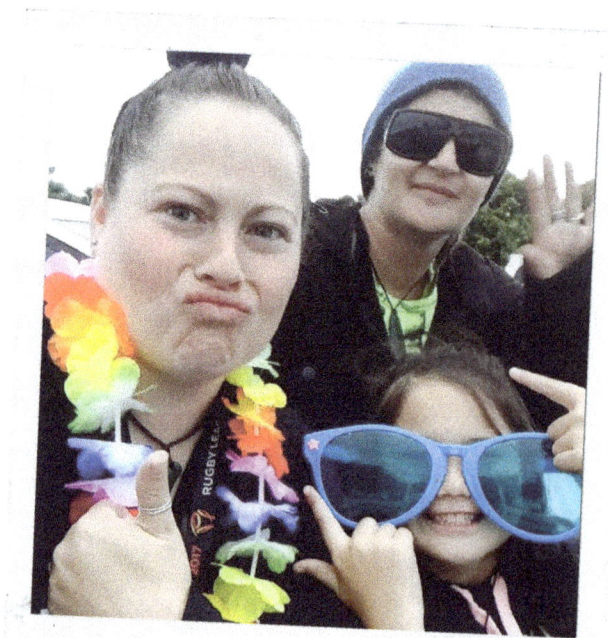

CREATE A LIFE YOU LOVE

Carrie Brightwell

Transformation and Growth

Transformation and growth are attainable when you learn how to take back your power, reconnect to yourself, discover your dreams and find a sense of purpose so that you can take the path towards a life you choose.

Here I have listed a few simple activities you can do to help you along that path.

Take back your power:
Power is metaphysical, meaning it exists (as energy) but you can't materialistically measure it. When you have power you can create and manifest. There are many ways in which we give our power away or it is taken from us. For example, not choosing what flavour ice cream I want and allowing someone else to decide for me is giving away my power. Equally, following the social narrative and doing the 'norm' is giving away power. Someone telling me I can't keep my job unless I sign a contract to say I will work on Saturdays is taking my power. The same can be said for a parent telling you that you were no good at something. In these cases, the other person or institution has your power, and whilst they have that energy you don't feel powerful. So, you don't have courage or creativity or drive or enthusiasm. To create a life we love we have to take back the energy that is ours so that we can feel, think, and dream from a place of power.

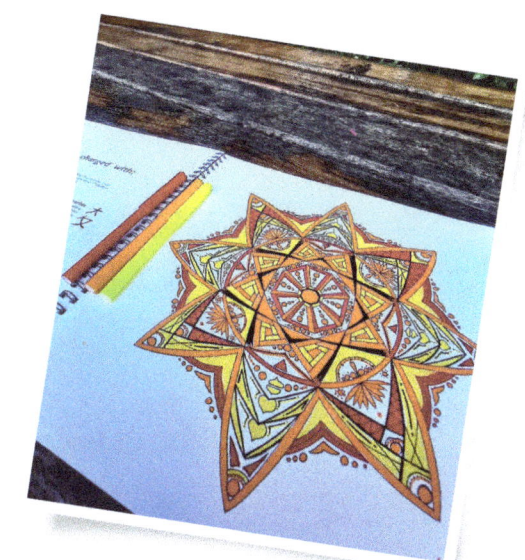

Here's a simple meditation:
- Get comfy, close your eyes and take some deep breaths to let the mind and body relax.
- See yourself standing in nature, take a stick and draw a circle on the ground around you.
- Imagine the person/institution you gave your power to or who took it, standing on the other side of that line. They cannot cross it.
- Demand that your power is returned to you. Watch as this energy comes back to you. Don't force the vision, just allow it to come as it wants to.
- If the person/institution struggles to give it back - take it.
- Once all the power has returned, send them on their way.
- Open your eyes when you feel ready to.
- Repeat this process as many times as necessary.

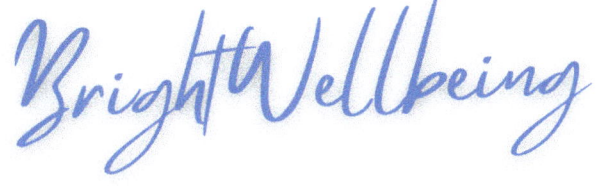

Carrie Brightwell

CREATE A LIFE YOU LOVE

Reconnect to Yourself

You have all of the answers inside of you. You just need to create the time and space to be able to connect to your true inner voice and feelings.

- Nature - spending time in nature, in solitude and without distraction (earphones, books etc), helps you to connect to the oneness that is you. So that you can hear your thoughts and feel your emotions. You can learn more about the positive impact of nature https://www.youtube.com/watch?v=iZpHJt1LKY4
- Love List - Write a list of 20 things that you love and do a minimum of 3 of them every single day. This helps you to know yourself and create boundaries. If you can't think of 20 then you create a Curiosity list, a list of the things you're curious to try. Exploring these will help you to get to yourself better. Learn more and download your free lists https://brightwellbeing.co.uk/your-love-list-curiosity-lists

Discover Your Dreams:

- Daydream - when was the last time you allowed yourself to daydream about what you truly want? We can only manifest that which we can see with our mind's eye and visualisation is like a muscle we need to strengthen. Allow yourself to regularly daydream about the future experience of life you want.

- Consider:
  - How do you want to feel every day?
  - What is your lifestyle?
  - Where do you want to be?
  - What do you want to be doing?
  - Who are you with?
  - What can you see, hear, smell, touch?
- Meditation - take the time to regularly put yourself into a meditative state so that you can see the wanderings of the mind and princess your thoughts/emotions.

Find a Sense of Purpose:

Your purpose is not something you can figure out with the mind, you need to feel your way to your purpose. Consider things like:

- What are you doing when you feel most alive?
- What are you doing when you get the most recognition, praise and value?
- What are known to be good at or for within your community/family/friends?

Use purpose reflection journal prompts to help you feel your way to your purpose. You can receive monthly purpose reflection journal prompts as part of my membership. Find out more https://brightwellbeing.co.uk/membership

INSPIRATION & MOTIVATION
BY MEGAN GALLAGHER

What inspires you to walk into your classroom every day?

What motivates you to keep learning and growing as a kaiako?

How do your ākonga inspire you?

Taking a moment to reflect on what inspires and motivates you is a powerful way to reconnect with your purpose and passion for teaching. Every day, you bring energy and care to your ākonga, but where does that drive come from?

Reflect on the moments that light a spark in you – the smiles, the 'aha' moments from ākonga, or the joy of seeing them grow and learn.

Are there specific professional goals, ideas, or challenges that push you to become better at your craft?

Think about the unique personalities, the curiosity and the resilience of your ākonga. How do they shape your teaching?

Reflect on the strategies, personal values, or support systems that help you stay motivated when things get challenging.

Whether it's seeing your ākonga thrive or creating a supportive learning environment, what drives you to care for their holistic well-being?

Taking stock of what currently inspires and motivates you, you're refueling your passion and purpose. Share your reflections with your colleagues or whānau and celebrate what makes you a kaiako who leads with heart and commitment.

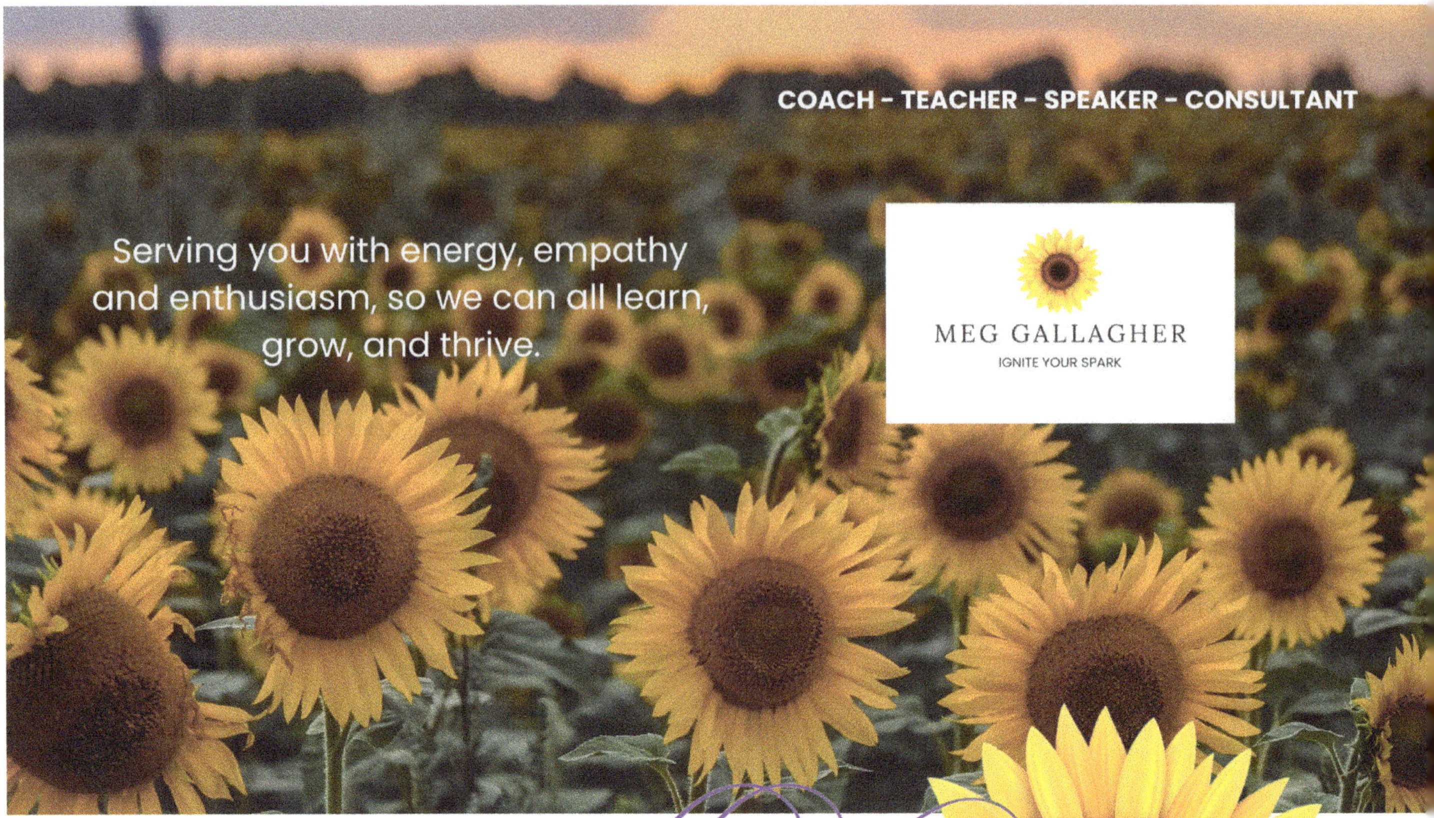

COACH – TEACHER – SPEAKER – CONSULTANT

Serving you with energy, empathy and enthusiasm, so we can all learn, grow, and thrive.

MEG GALLAGHER
IGNITE YOUR SPARK

Meg Gallagher

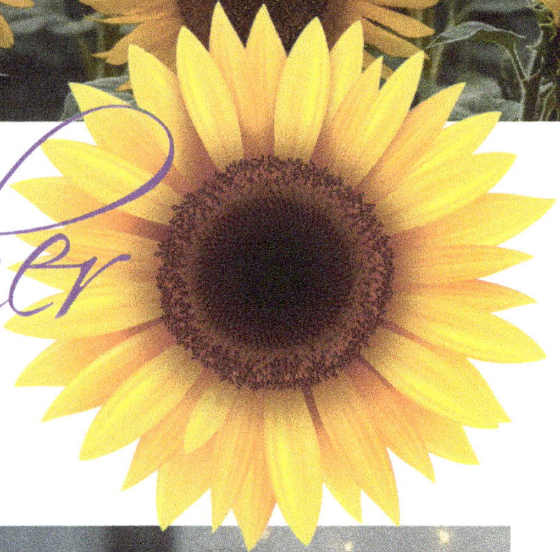

Contact me:
Website: https://www.meggallagher.nz/

Email: meg@meggallagher.nz

Follow me and join in the conversations:
Substack: Writing to support and inspire educators.
https://heartandbraininmind.substack.com

Happy Healthy Teachers Matter FB Group:
A positive place for teacher wellbeing support.
https://www.facebook.com/share/g/1AZ5HDyvL6

FB Page: Teaching and Learning inspiration and support.
www.facebook.com/teachingwithheartandbraininmind

Teacher Wellbeing research link:
A summary of my masters research.
https://nzareblog.wordpress.com/2017/12/06/teacher-wellbeing

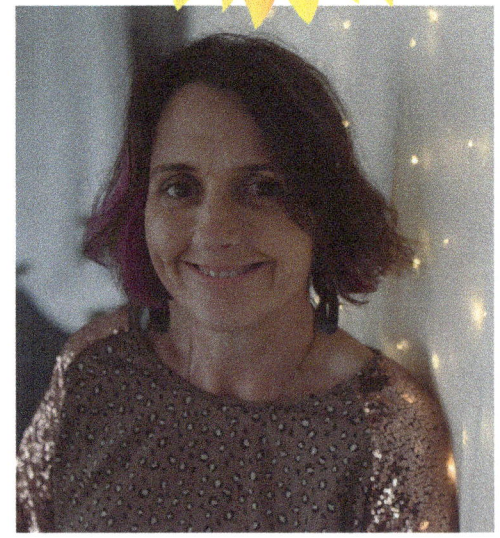

Kia ora koutou,
Ko Kaitangata te whenua tipu engari ko Palmerston, Otago, tōhoku kaika inanianei.
Ko Megan Gallagher ahau.
He hākui me he kaiako ahau.
Nō reira, tēnā koutou katoa.

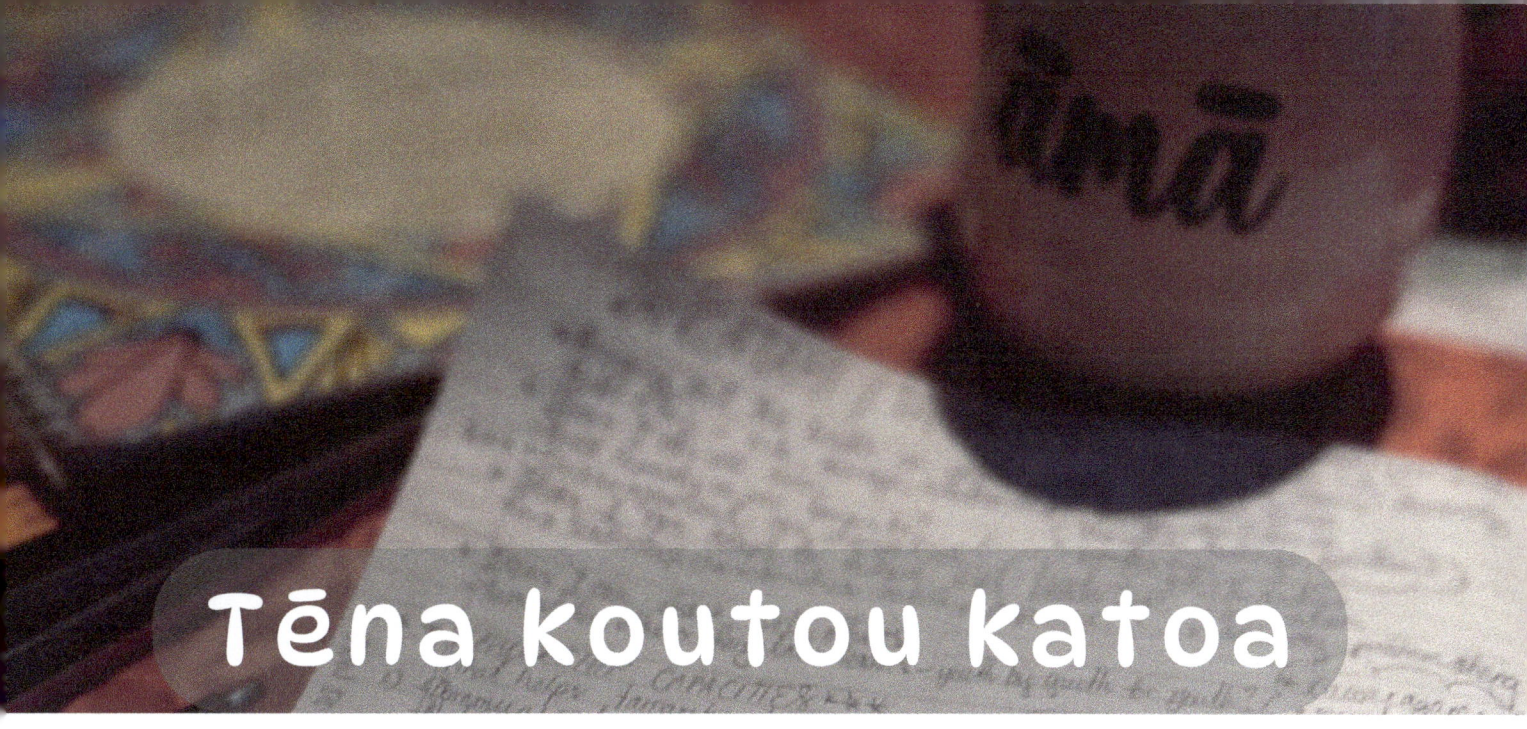

Tēna koutou katoa

To Our Kaiako, Kaimahi, Kaiawhina

You carry the future on your shoulders, guiding our tamariki mokopuna with patience, with care that stretches beyond the day, into the nights of preparation and quiet reflection.

Your hands shape more than lessons, they shape confidence, culture and a sense of belonging—nurturing minds to grow and hearts to feel proud.

In every challenge, you offer strength, in every pātai, you offer understanding and in every moment of doubt, you offer the gift of believing in them, even when they cannot yet see it themselves.

You are the harakeke inter-woven with wisdom, kindness and aroha. For this, we thank you. Ngā mihi for your tireless energy, for standing by their side, for making space for their dreams to take flight.

Ngā mihi nui ki a koutou katoa,
for all that you do,
for all that you are,
for all that you give.

Whakawhetai, whakawhetai, whakawhetai.

End of Pukapuka Gratitude

As we wrap up this pukapuka, I want to take a moment to express my heartfelt gratitude to the incredible people who have supported me throughout this haerenga and for those who have picked this pukapuka up and put it down and picked it up again.

To my whānau and friends who encouraged me when I needed it the most. Thank you also for helping me prioritise my hauora while bringing *Oranga* to life. It has been a privilege having you walk this journey with me. May we continue to prioritise our wellbeing.

Kaiako mā, your hard work doesn't go unnoticed. Your energy, kindness and commitment you bring every day is appreciated by many.

Taking on the learnings, building our confidence and working together, we can make a positive impact, not only in the lives of our ākonga, also within your own teams.

Here's to recharging each day, not hanging out for the weekend - every day, so we can keep going and coming back stronger, refreshed and ready to continue making a difference! 💛

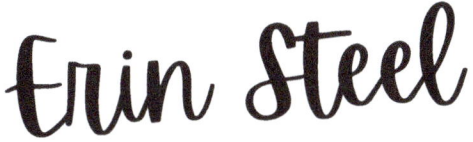

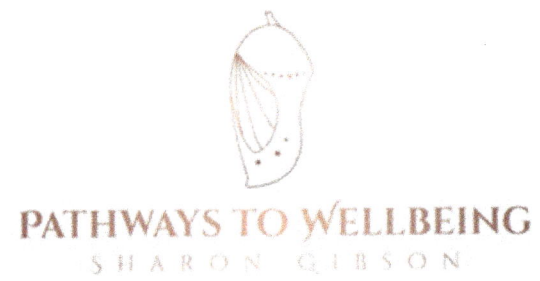

PATHWAYS TO WELLBEING
SHARON GIBSON

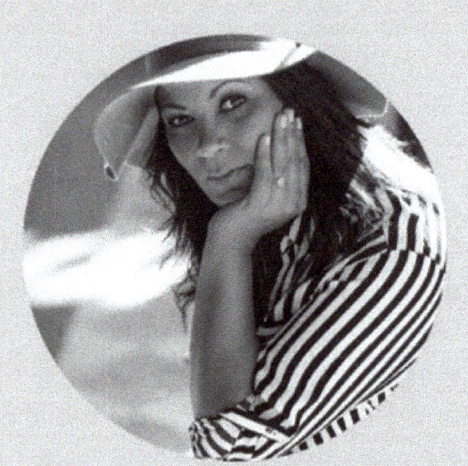

Hi, I'm Sharon, an accredited Mental Health First Aid Aotearoa Instructor

As a mental health first aid instructor, my main aim is to establish a safe, supportive, and non-judgmental environment for trainees. I aim to empower them with the knowledge and confidence to spot the symptoms, and address individuals facing mental health challenges or crises until necessary assistance is received. Drawing from my extensive lived experience and 13 years of Wellbeing Facilitation, I provide valuable insights to those I work with.

MHFA is an international training adapted to meet the cultural needs of Aotearoa. Te Pou, part of the Wise Group, holds the license to deliver this education in NZ.

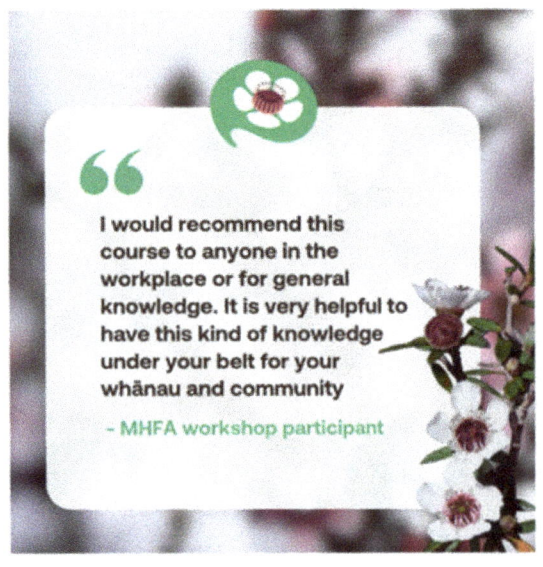

"I would recommend this course to anyone in the workplace or for general knowledge. It is very helpful to have this kind of knowledge under your belt for your whānau and community

- MHFA workshop participant

Why attend a Mental Health First Aid course?

MHFA training enhances understanding, confidence, and early intervention for mental health challenges, reducing stigma and discrimination. Early intervention prevents long term recovery.

Who can attend the course?
Anyone over 18 can attend the course.
NB: This is not a therapy or support group.

www.pathwaystowellbeing.co.nz   Mob: 0212 442 811   hello@pathwaystowellbeing.co.nz

ACKNOWLEDGEMENTS

Writing this book has been an incredible haerenga,
And I am deeply grateful for all those who have supported me along the way.

Whakawhetai tuatahi, to my whānau—
Nathan, my husband, Jaxon Maniah and Wiremu Kahurangi, our tamariki.
Your endless aroha, patience and encouragement—
You are my inspiration, my strength.
Thank you for the time, the space and for believing in my dream.

Whakawhetai tuarua, to my mum Carol and my sister Kat—
For nurturing my love of learning, of stories, of books.
Since as far back as I can remember, you have given me the awhi I've needed,
You've guided me with aroha and believed in me,
Shaping who I am today. I am forever grateful.

Whakawhetai tuatoru, to Karen Tui Boyes,
My editor, mentor, friend and gratitude sister.
Your expert insight and trust in my vision—
Since the beginning, you've helped bring this book to life.

Whakawhetai tuawhā, to my mentors and teachers—
Meg Gallagher, Carrie Brightwell—
Your wisdom, knowledge and belief in me have carried me far.
Rangi Neho, Alysha Howie, Jen Fielden, Natalie Wilcock and Jessie Patch—
Thank you for reading, for feedback, for your ongoing encouragement,
For helping refine this work when I needed it most.

To my hoamahi at Sport Northland—
In our Healthy Active Learning team, you inspire me every day.
Your passion and commitment to Te Tai Tokerau are the heart of this book.

And finally, to you, the reader—
Thank you for taking this journey with me.
I hope these words uplift you, as writing them has uplifted me.

Ngā mihi nui ki a koutou katoa.
Erin Steel

Testimonials:

I am beyond proud to call Erin tōku hoa, my friend. Her heart is huge and I am so thrilled to see what she has created here for kaiako. This pukapuka is a guide that will support us all to care for ourselves and our energy. Our oranga and hauora are taonga that enable us to make a positive difference in the lives of the people we work and play with.
Kā mihi nui, Erin, tōku hoa for all that you give the communities you care for.
Megan Gallagher

This book is just one of the examples of the sunshine Erin shares with the world. Throughout my time of working with Erin as a teacher, and becoming her friend and work colleague, she has inspired, taught, supported, and spread joy to me and others in her circles. Erins commitment to helping others, through her own personal experiences and learnings and the lens of hauora over everything she thinks about, has led her to craft this book to help kaiako, who I know she thinks are some of the greatest and most valuable people in our world. Erin is a dedicated learner and a true queen of manaakitanga. She is a valued colleague and friend, and loves a lemon honey and ginger drink!
Jen Fielden

Testimonials:

Oranga - Mental Health Matters, is an outstanding resource, offering an engaging and comprehensive approach to the well-being of Kaiako and their students. This work by Erin Steel is thoughtfully designed, using her 20 years of teaching experience and passion for mental health matters, to provide practical strategies and insights that align with the unique needs of Kaiako here in Aotearoa New Zealand. Erin's expertise is on display, with advice on managing stress, building resilience, and creating positive, supportive learning environments. Erin incorporates Māori perspectives and values throughout her work, highlighting the importance of cultural values and practises in Aotearoa New Zealand's diverse educational landscape. The addition of Erin's personal poetry peppers the pages with her own examples of meditation and moments of reflection. This essential resource is a powerful tool which can help Kaiako navigate the challenges of their role while maintaining their own well-being.
Rangi Neho

I am truly grateful for this pukapuka. With offerings of guidance it not only reminds us of the importance of taking care of our mental health but provides practical and achievable tips and strategies to do so. He oranga ngākau, he pikinga wairua' this book truely touches my heart and lifts my spirits. When people thrive, the world thrives, when our kaiako thrive, so do our tamariki. I highly recommend this resource to all kaiako who are dedicated to nurturing a healthy mind and to those who want to make a start!
Jessie Patch

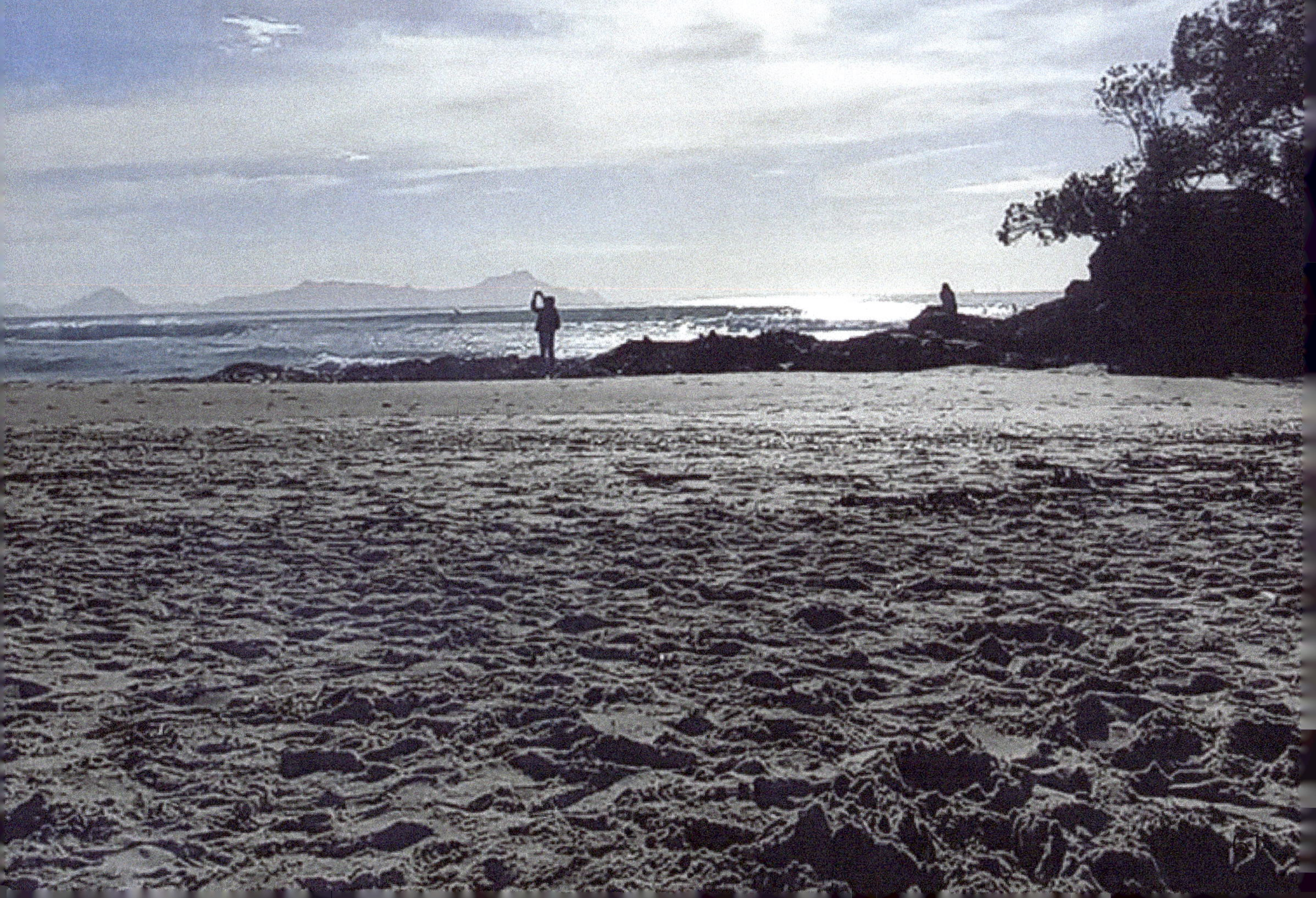

www.ingramcontent.com/pod-product-compliance
Lightning Source LLC
Chambersburg PA
CBHW041657040426
R18086800001B/R180868PG42333CBX00005B/1